DINESH BHUGRA

GW00496515

Mental Heath
of Ethnic Minorities

An Annotated Bibliography

GASKELL

© The Royal College of Psychiatrists 1999

Gaskell is an imprint and registered trade mark of the Royal College of Psychiatrists, 17 Belgrave Square, London SW1X 8PG

Gaskell and the College crest are registered trade marks of the Royal College of Psychiatrists.

All rights reserved. No part of this book may be reprinted or reproduced or utilised in any form or by any electronic, mechanical, or other means, now known or hereafter invented, including photocopying and recording, or in any information storage or retrieval system, without permission in writing from the publishers.

British Library Cataloguing-in-Publication Data
A catalogue record for this book is available from the British Library.
ISBN 1-901242-31-5

Distributed in North America
by American Psychiatric Press, Inc.
ISBN 0-88048-599-X

The views presented in this book do not necessarily reflect those of the Royal College of Psychiatrists, and the publishers are not responsible for any error of omission or fact.

The Royal College of Psychiatrists is a registered charity (no. 228636).

Cover design by The Graphic Group, West Sussex
Printed by Bell & Bain Limited, Glasgow

Contents

Preface

Over the past 20 years there has been an increased interest in the mental health needs of minority ethnic groups in the UK. This has led to a body of research, both epidemiological and anthropological, which has often been criticised for simplifying specific issues to do with ethnic minority mental health. Over the years, researchers have become increasingly aware of the problems of definition, data collection, survey design as well as interpretation of the findings. Increasingly, communities themselves are being involved in planning and carrying out research as well as helping researchers to interpret findings. Another welcome development has been the role of voluntary organisations which have provided support for and sometimes even carried out research, as well as lobbying to influence social policy.

The collection of research papers annotated here have been selected because they report work which has been novel, and sometimes controversial, and have a contribution to make to both clinical service delivery and research. They come largely from within the UK. No attempt has been made to be fully comprehensive – the purpose of the book is to provide an introduction to researchers, mental health professionals and other health care delivery personnel who are interested in this field. The aim is to stimulate future research and thinking on the topic and to point the reader in the right direction for further reading. Some terms (although unacceptable now) have been left in place to reflect the accuracy of the research as well as to highlight historical changes in the use and misuse of some terms.

I am grateful to Ms Veena Bahl, at the Department of Health, for securing funding for publication of this volume, and without whose help, guidance and support this project would never have taken off. I am also thankful to Caroline Harding and Rachel Lippett, among others, for their hard work.

Dinesh Bhugra
London

Executive summary

Background

1. Black and minority populations form approximately 6% of the population of England and Wales. Most of these populations are concentrated in large metropolitan cities.
2. The recent white papers and the green paper on *Modernising Health Services* and *Our Healthier Nation* provide an opportunity to examine mental health in the context of providing a seamless approach to health and social care.
3. These reports provide a useful way forward in determining the causes of mental illness, including social determinants such as poverty and unemployment.
4. The social and economic status of Black and minority ethnic groups may influence their presentation, which will determine pathways into care and help-seeking, both at primary and at secondary care levels.
5. There is some evidence that there are delays in help-seeking and individuals from some minority groups may well seek help from alternative sources prior to approaching statutory services.

Recent research

1. Rates of different mental illnesses vary across different ethnic groups. For example, inception rates of schizophrenia have been shown to be consistently higher among African–Carribeans when compared with some other ethnic groups. These rates are said to be higher among siblings of those diagnosed as having schizophrenia, thereby suggesting that a range of factors may well be at play.
2. Earlier studies had demonstrated that rates of admission of Asians to psychiatric hospital were higher than those of the indigenous populations, suggesting that levels and rates of illness were higher; however, the pathways to care are influenced by other factors including severity and accessibility to services. The findings have not been consistent.
3. The rates of mental illness among Black prisoners have been shown to be higher than in White prisoners. The reasons for such differences include differential rates of offending, past psychiatric history and poor contact with psychiatric services.

4. Drinking patterns vary across different ethnic groups. For example, Black and White subjects drink similar amounts but Sikhs show much higher than expected rates of drinking.
5. The rates of compulsory detention have been shown to be higher among some ethnic groups, although these findings are not consistent and appear to influence first contact as well as subsequent admissions.
6. Inception rates of deliberate self-harm are not higher among Asian adolescents, but are definitely higher among Asian females over the age of 18 compared with Whites, suggesting that social factors come into play in this age group as well as level of functioning. Asian women are also more likely to commit suicide by burning.
7. Developing and using culture-specific tools to screen dementias may well identify unmet needs across different communities. There are clear differences across different ethnic groups in the way in which distress is expressed, especially in the context of common mental disorders such as anxiety and depression.
8. The inception rates of mania are not increased among Black and ethnic minority groups.
9. The increased rate of schizophrenia among African–Caribbeans has been shown not to be related to biological factors like pregnancy and birth complications.
10. Black Caribbean patients have been shown to be more dissatisfied than their White counterparts with the statutory services. This has been shown to be related to number of previous admissions.

The future

1. The reasons for high rates of schizophrenia among African–Caribbeans need to be investigated using epidemiological, biological and qualitative methods.
2. The cultural and social factors contributing to increased rates of attempted suicide in Asian females and completed suicide by burning need to be investigated.
3. Culturally sensitive screening instruments need to be developed to screen common mental disorders and dementias across different ethnic groups.
4. To reduce dissatisfaction, services must be developed in a culturally sensitive, culturally acceptable and accessible manner, and the communities must be involved in service planning.

Abas, M. (1996) Depression and anxiety among older Caribbean people in the UK: screening, unmet need and the provision of appropriate services. *International Journal of Geriatric Psychiatry*, **11**, 377–382.

Introduction

Despite the fact that increasing numbers of older people living in the UK are members of ethnic minorities, little has been written about depression and anxiety among them. Recent changes in monitoring requirements have meant that comprehensive health service data according to ethnicity are now available. However, myths that, for example, ethnic minority elders are always cared for within extended family networks or that they are more likely to somatise symptoms of depression have had a negative impact. Controversy also exits in relation to the actual distribution of these problems in ethnic minority communities. What is clear, the author of the paper points out, are the negative perceptions of statutory mental health services held by the Black community.

This paper describes the development of a new culture-specific tool for screening anxiety and depression in Caribbean elders and discusses its usefulness in identifying unmet need and appropriate services. The Royal College of General Practitioners recommends the use of the Geriatric Depression Scale (GDS) to screen for emotional distress; however, doubts exist about its reliability when used in relation to ethnic minority elders. The new culture-specific screen for use with older Caribbean people, developed by Professor Raymond Levy and others at the Institute of Psychiatry (see Abas *et al*, 1996, below), may be more effective. In a recent community pilot study using the new scale, 17% of a random sample of Caribbean elders were found to be experiencing emotional distress – half of whom met the DSM–III–R criteria for depression. Two-thirds of the others in the sample were seen by their families and a Caribbean nurse as being severely 'stressed' and needing help.

The development of the culture-specific screen

Non-psychiatrically trained carers (e.g. church ministers, voluntary workers and home carers) and elders identified by them as being emotionally distressed were interviewed and the results used to generate a lay Caribbean classification of mental illness. Over 100 idioms linked to non-psychotic distress were identified, and these were grouped into 13 domains such as worrying/fretting, feeling low or down, feeling pressured, feeling empty inside and so on. (The word 'depression' was mentioned by only 9% of respondents.) Idioms from these 13 domains were used to create the preliminary screen.

One way in which the new screen differed from the GDS and others was in the inclusion of concepts such as feeling 'cut off' or 'fed up' – symptoms identified by Caribbeans that were not included in previous screens. Also, the concept of 'emptiness' in the GDS relates to a person's life being empty – but Caribbean elders tended to emphasise a personal sense of emptiness.

It appears that the screen distinguished well between cases of depression and non-depression. However, the author acknowledges problems in using definitions of 'caseness' for Caribbean elders based on medical psychiatric assessment rather than notions of abnormality based on the assessment of the Caribbean community. At the time of writing, a full-scale validation exercise, based on a consensus of key Black Caribbean professionals, was under way.

Unmet need

The author highlights the difficulty general practitioners have assessing mental illness in members of ethnic minorities. We are told that in a recent pilot survey all the depressed Caribbean elders identified had unmet needs and that many of these were subsequently addressed using existing health and social care services – some services were viewed by the community as inappropriate. The author highlights the need to investigate communities' attitudes to depression in order to find out whether services are accessible and appropriate.

The use of an exploratory model, taking account of people's own views about their illness and treatment, when assessing need, is recommended in addition to formal needs assessment. Comparing the results of the 'professional' instrument with the views of patients and carers is also suggested. The preference of ethnic minority elders in relation to the way in which services are delivered, it is said, also needs investigation.

Abas, M., Phillips, C., Richards, M., Carter, J. & Levy, R. (1996) Initial development of a new culture-specific screen for emotional distress in older Caribbean people. *International Journal of Geriatric Psychiatry*, **11**, 1097–1103.

Introduction

Consultations for depression and anxiety are lower among ethnic minority elders than for the White population. Ethnic minority elders are also under-represented among patients using community and hospital mental health services. The Geriatric Depression Scale (GDS), recommended by the Royal College of General Practitioners, has not been validated for use with Caribbean elders. Evidence suggests differences exist in the way people from different cultures express and experience depression and anxiety. Older Caribbeans, for example, speak of being 'low spirited', 'fed up' and 'weighted down'. This paper reports the development of a new culture-specific screen, based on the way in which Caribbean elders express feelings of emotional distress.

Method

The screen went through several stages of development. The first involved the development of a mental disorder classification system. Twenty-one community figures (such as church ministers, day care and residential workers, Black users' representatives and so on) from 12 organisations working with Caribbean elders took part in interviews and focus groups. Most of the community figures had their roots in Jamaica, the rest coming from other areas of the Caribbean. The most commonly described lay mental illness categories were: being stressed out; having a depressed spirit; and senility and madness – believing things about themselves which were not true or saying things had happened which had not.

Stage 2 of the development involved gathering terms to describe emotional distress in Caribbean elders. Participants were asked to expand on the common symptoms and terms detected at stage 1, and to identify elders suffering from these symptoms. Fourteen such elders were consequently identified and 11 of them agreed to be interviewed. A content analysis of Caribbean literature was also carried out to find other terms for emotional distress. A total of 119 terms were identified.

Stage 3 involved the development of a preliminary culture-specific screen. Here the terms were grouped into 23 domains by experienced Caribbean professionals, who included a social worker, a sociologist, a psychiatric nurse and two pastors. Using a consensus approach, idioms from what were determined to be the 12 key domains were chosen to create the preliminary screening tool.

Stage 4 involved piloting the screen. This was done in three parts. First, a community register of local Caribbean residents aged over 65 years was developed by knocking on doors in one of the electoral wards of the London Borough of Southwark. Eighty elders were identified, of whom 35 took part in both a health screening interview and a psychiatric assessment. In the second part of the pilot study, 18 Caribbean elders, known to local community or hospital mental health workers, were questioned. In the third part, 10 subjects, identified by Caribbean church pastors and workers from three voluntary day centres as not coping with stress or suffering from a depressed spirit, were questioned. The screen, used by both Caribbean and non-Caribbean interviewers, was acceptable to respondents and the reliability of the screen was found to be high.

Stage 5 of the development involved the addition of an extra item to the screen as a result of the community data. This item, fearful or palpitating heart, had been identified previously but not given high priority.

Discussion

The researchers found that the term 'depression' was hardly used and 'suicidal intent' not at all. While a comparison of the screen with commonly used non-culture specific ones showed some overlap in terms, there were some differences. For example, the feeling of being 'cut off' was found in 70% of depressed Caribbean cases identified. The item concerning feeling 'fed up' was one of the most common idioms used but it was not part of the two most widely used scales. The results of the investigation were in line with culture-specific expressions of depression reported by other researchers – for example, feeling low, feeling tired, and having pains all over.

The inclusion of items commonly associated with anxiety, such as sensation of gas bubbling in the stomach, led the authors to suggest that the screen would detect the common forms of depression found in primary care as these tend to be associated with anxiety. The necessity of a full-scale validation is acknowledged and this was in progress at the time the paper was written.

Ananthanarayanan, T. S. (1994) Epidemiology of mental illness among Asians in the UK. *British Journal of Hospital Medicine,* **52,** 500–506.

Introduction

This paper highlights the fact that researchers interested in the rate of psychiatric illness in immigrants from the Indian subcontinent often forget to take into account the fact that a significant number of immigrants from India are of White British origin. Mental health and ethnicity studies are reviewed with this point in mind.

Review

While migration has been linked to increased rates of psychiatric disorder, epidemiological studies of psychiatric morbidity have produced conflicting results. Schizophrenia is the most common diagnosis in both Indian-born and Pakistani-born immigrant groups. However, the author suggests caution is needed when considering this information because of the difficulties inherent in diagnosing schizophrenia in patients whose first language is not English.

The studies reviewed show no significant differences in rates of admission for affective disorder among Asian immigrants as compared with the White British-born population. They do, however, highlight the prominence of somatic symptoms among the Asian UK population. There is also a significantly higher rate of admission for alcoholism reported among Indians. Studies have shown higher rates of hysterical dissociation symptoms among young Asian women, something that is relatively rare in the West. Asian women also have higher rates of attempted suicide and deliberate self-harm. However, community surveys have tended to show relatively low rates of psychiatric morbidity among Asians, particularly the Indian population.

Anumonye, A. (1967) Psychological stresses among African students in Britain. *Scottish Medical Journal,* **12,** 314–319.

African students attending universities in the UK suffering from mental health problems were more likely to be female, from a non-Western cultural background, and experiencing financial problems and problems with language. The author suggests that African students have, on the one hand, some universal problems such as colour discrimination, climatic factors, poor accommodation, separation reaction, language problems, sexual difficulties, restricted choices, disillusionment, poor adjustment, dietary problems; and, on the other, British peculiarities such as proverbial coldness and inhibition and loneliness. Unaccommodating social values in the country of origin – which means that the academically unsuccessful students are unwilling to return home – and lack of a friendly reception in the host country also contribute to a sense of alienation and isolation.

The author also highlights other problems that African students face in this country. The suggestion that paranoid features, which are common as a form of reaction among both Westernised and non-Westernised African students, are related to a belief in magical phenomenon deserves to be studied further. Such an observation has provoked some Euro-American social psychologists to presume that African people are incapable of concept formation, which according to the author is not a sensible assumption. In addition to financial problems, poor preparation prior to migration and unexpected events all contribute to a sense of alienation.

The author mentions additional problems of a sexual nature where African students are said to be less inhibited than their British counterparts but more frightened by overt street-corner sexual behaviour. Their high visibility by virtue of their skin colour and prejudice may affect their functioning in university settings.

The best way to deal with the constellation of psychological problems of African students is embodied in the techniques of preventive psychiatry. The day-to-day social, academic and psychological problems can be helped by psychological and social intervention, including educating the student and others. The initial contact is of great importance for establishing confidence. The local health professionals must be made aware of different presentations, precipitating factors and management strategies.

Banerjee, S., O'Neill-Byrne, K., Exworthy, T. & Parrott, J. (1995) The Belmarsh Scheme – a prospective study of the transfer of mentally disordered remand prisoners from prison to psychiatric units. *British Journal of Psychiatry*, **166**, 802–805.

Introduction

Reports published by the Department of Health and the Home Office support the purchase from the National Health Service, by prisons, of psychiatric services for mentally disordered offenders, in order to improve their mental health care. However, few such schemes have been set up, and before this study no evaluation of such a scheme had been published. This piece evaluates the 'Belmarsh Scheme', which operates in south London.

Method

Researchers investigated all prisoners remanded in custody to Her Majesty's Prison Belmarsh during a six-month period in 1992. All prisoners were medically screened upon reception into the prison;

some were then admitted to the health care centre, where they were then given a full psychiatric assessment. Forensic and general consultant supervisors reached a joint decision with the prison-based psychiatrists as to which prisoners required a transfer to psychiatric services. For those who were to be transferred, demographic data, details of the alleged offence, details of contact with psychiatric services and diagnosis (using DSM–III–R) were also collected, and compared with the characteristics of all other prisoners remanded to prison during the six-month period under study.

Results

Of the 1229 new remands, 53 were transferred to psychiatric units. Of these, 77% had been psychiatric in-patients previously, but only 34% were receiving psychiatric help at the time of their arrest. Every patient who was deemed to require a transfer *was* transferred. Forty per cent were admitted to open wards, 34% to locked wards, 21% to regional secure units, and 2% to special hospitals. There was a significantly higher proportion of Black men in the group transferred in comparison with all other remand prisoners. Among all those transferred, the mean length of time spent in prison was 32.6 days (range 2–130 days).

Discussion

The authors state that their research illustrates that considerable numbers of severely mentally ill men are remanded into custody. Although they state that their study did not aim to address the reasons why Black men are disproportionately represented in this group, they suggest a number of possible explanations (including higher rates of mental disorder within this group, or a possible differential rate of offending) and call for this finding to be investigated urgently. The authors go on to detail other studies where large numbers of prisoners who were assessed as requiring psychiatric help were subsequently refused treatment, and use this evidence to suggest that the Belmarsh Scheme was more effective in ensuring that those who required treatment did in fact receive it. The researchers draw attention to the fact that 77% of transferred prisoners had been psychiatric in-patients, but that only one-third were under psychiatric care at the time of their arrest and state that perhaps if contact with psychiatric services had been maintained, a relapse of illness could have been prevented.

Bhatnagar, K. & Frank, J. (1997) Psychiatric disorders in elderly from the Indian sub-continent living in Bradford. *International Journal of Geriatric Psychiatry*, **12**, 907–912.

Introduction

The authors set out to study rates of psychiatric disorders in elderly people originating from the Indian subcontinent living in Bradford.

Method

They identified Asian names supplied by the Family Health Service Authority and selected every fifth subject. The subjects were contacted by letter initially, and using Hindi translations of the Geriatric Mental State Examination they were interviewed and a clinical psychiatric diagnosis given. Of a total population of 1065 elderly Asians, 213 contacts were derived. Fourteen had to be excluded. Of the 199 remaining, 97 could not be contacted, one refused and another one was hospitalised, thus 100 interviews were completed.

Results

Of 100 interviewees, 25% were living alone (including 15% in sheltered housing) and the rest with their spouses or children. Three quarters (74%) were male. The age range was from 65–89 years. The total prevalence of psychiatric disorder was 28% (CI 19.4%– 37.07%) according to psychiatric diagnosis and 29% (CI 20.36%–38.03%) according to GMS–AGECAT. Prevalence of depression was 20% according to both criteria, neurotic disorders 4% and organic disorders (dementia) 4%.

The high prevalence of depression in this sample is higher than predicted and may be attributed to additional social problems. The authors suggest a constitutional vulnerability and also additional physical health problems. The sample was predominantly male suggesting that other factors may be at play. The authors also observed a lack of guilt feelings and suicidal ideas in this group. GMS–AGECAT did not often pick up diagnosis of dementia but the psychiatrist did so, and the questionnaire may well have an educational and cultural bias.

Discussion

In spite of the high attrition rates of subjects, the reason being that many subjects had either moved or were abroad, the study highlights high rates of depression and low rates of dementia in Asian elderly subjects. A lack of control group, however, makes the study's findings of limited significance.

Bhugra, D. & Bhui, K. (1997) Cross cultural psychiatric assessment. *Advances in Psychiatric Treatment*, **3**, 103–110.

Bhugra, D. & Bhui, K. (1997) Clinical management of patients across cultures. *Advances in Psychiatric Treatment*, **3**, 233–239

Bhugra, D. & Bhui, K. (1999) Ethnic and cultural factors in psychopharmacology. *Advances in Psychiatric Treatment*, **5**, 89–95.

In these three papers the authors provide a theoretical overview on the assessment, management and pharmacological treatment of patients from different cultures.

In the first paper, the authors define the relationships between culture and mental illness and the role of cultural competencies for clinicians. The methods of setting up clinical assessment are described along with the assessment of migration and the importance of world view, adverse events and acculturation in the assessment. The limitations of the standard mental state examination are described along with recommendations for assessing explanatory models of illness. The authors suggest that sensitivity and clinical assessment go hand in hand.

In the second paper, principles of management are defined. These include identifying the goals of treatment, planning treatment and implementing a pharmacotherapy plan. The roles of electro-convulasive therapy, complementary therapies, indigenous therapies and psychotherapy, including cognitive techniques, are described. Methods of confrontation without threat are illustrated and management and service development are discussed.

In the third paper, personality and environmental factors – especially biological factors – are described in relation to psycho-pharmacology. Pharmacokinetics and pharmacodynamics are defined and differences in these across ethnic groups are illustrated with specific examples of various psychiatric drugs. Non-biological factors like stress, availability of drugs and prescription patterns are discussed along with the role of complementary medicine.

Discussion

These three papers provide a theoretical overview in assessing and managing patients whose culture and ethnicity differs from that of the therapists.

Bhugra, D., Baldwin, D. & Desai, M. (1997) Focus groups: implications for primary and cross-cultural psychiatry. *Primary Care Psychiatry*, **3**, 45–50.

In this paper, the authors illustrate the need for qualitative data collection in cross-cultural and primary care psychiatry. The goal of qualitative research is the development of concepts that help us to understand social phenomena in natural settings. The meanings, experiences and views of the participants are given due emphasis and representation. The methodological rigour of qualitative research is as important. The role of the emic (culture-specific) method of data collection and recognising relativism of cultures are important factors in setting up focus groups. The authors demonstrate these in a focus group of Punjabi women from west London. Using a case vignette of a depressed woman, the subjects were encouraged to discuss and comment on possible causative and management factors. They recognised symptoms of depression as excessive thinking, weight on mind, pressure on brain, poor concentration, poor sleep, forgetfulness, unwanted intrusive thoughts, excessive tiredness, restlessness, sadness, feeling of heat, poor appetite, low self-esteem and shame. Aetiological causes identified were family conflict, death, unemployment, financial difficulties and failure to succeed. Talking about problems was seen as very important and the use of religious activities was more relevant than going to their GP. The general attitude towards management was a preference for a non-medical self-reliant model. The authors describe the advantages and disadvantages of the focus groups.

Discussion

The observations cannot be applied across the board and more similar focus groups need to be conducted across different communities.

Bhugra, D., Leff, J., Mallett, R., Der, G., Corridan, B. & Rudge, S. (1997) Incidence and outcome of schizophrenia in whites, African-Caribbeans and Asians in London. *Psychological Medicine,* **27,** 791–798.

Introduction

Epidemiological studies investigating the incidence of schizophrenia among different ethnic communities have focused almost exclusively on African–Caribbeans, for whom higher rates are reported. The authors of the paper suggest that comparing rates among Asian patients, with their similar experiences to African–Caribbeans of migration, discrimination and so on, would help to explore some hypotheses regarding the aetiology of schizophrenia.

Method

Patients using services provided by two London health districts with similar socio-economic and population profiles were screened for possible participation in the research. (The districts in question were Ealing, with a relatively large Asian population, and South Southwark/ East Lambeth, with a relatively large African–Caribbean population.) To be included in the study patients had to have been resident in the relevant catchment area for at least six months, to present with overt psychotic symptoms or two abnormalities suggestive of psychosis, and to be experiencing their first ever contact with services. People with an organic cerebral disorder were excluded. White patients were recruited only from Ealing, as White patients from the other district were already the subject of research.

Patients who passed the initial screening were assessed using the Present State Examination (PSE). To supplement this, nearest relatives were also interviewed and general practitioners were contacted. Patients were monitored over a one-year follow-up period, during which the PSE was repeated if symptoms recurred.

Results

The study subjects were 38 White, 38 African–Caribbean and 24 Asian patients. In comparison with the White and African–Caribbean patients, more Asians were aged over 30, had been born abroad and were married (50%). More African–Caribbeans were unemployed than either of the two other groups.

A comparison of the overall standardised rates for schizophrenia showed that only the differences between the African–Caribbean and White groups were statistically significant. However, after allowing for the influence of age and gender, the effect of ethnic group on incidence, as a whole, became significant. The rate for African–Caribbeans was roughly twice that of Whites in three of the four age and gender subgroups. Differences in age and gender distribution made Asian and White comparisons difficult – incidence rates for women and older Asians were relatively high.

Ethnicity was found to exert the greatest effect on outcome: 60% of African–Caribbean, 17% of Asian and 24% of White patients in the study were classified as having a poor outcome. Unemployment and gender also had a significant effect on outcome – but the effect of unemployment disappeared when the effects of ethnicity were considered. Only the gender effect remained significant – men had a worse outcome.

Discussion

In keeping with previous studies, African–Caribbeans were found to have a greater risk of developing a first episode of schizophrenia than Whites. However, the difference was smaller than in other studies, perhaps because more accurate population data and structured interviews were used. Among Asians, a high rate of schizophrenia compared with the White population was found only for those aged over 30, and especially for women. The findings suggest that the factors involved in the aetiology of schizophrenia operate differently, over the life cycle, for people in different ethnic groups. Further investigations are recommended.

The authors propose that the greater relapse rate among African–Caribbeans suggests that factors affecting outcome differ from those affecting aetiology. Unemployment, which was significantly greater among African–Caribbeans, could, they say, be one factor influencing relapse. A genetic cause is thought unlikely because of the results of two epidemiological studies (one in Jamaica, the other in Trinidad) which did not find higher incidence rates in African–Caribbeans.

Bhui, K. & Bhugra, D. (1998) Training and supervision in effective cross-cultural mental health services. *Hospital Medicine*, **59**, 861–865.

For mental health professionals working in catchment areas with significant numbers of Black and minority ethnic groups, not only is adequate training required in order to deliver effective mental health services, but clinical supervision is very important as well. Although racism and prejudicial attitudes are discussed at length these do not form part of any curriculum for training or supervision.

The authors describe three models of training and suggest that trainees can come from a number of sources including the voluntary sector and can be individuals, groups or organisations. Theoretical models of training are self-reflexive, experiential, behavioural–motivational or cognitive. They argue that culture should be an integral part of service development and training, and supervision must be inclusive in the processes of service development. Clinical supervision is mandatory for virtually all trainees but the interactions between the patient's and the therapist's world views are further complicated by the world view of the supervisor. Such interactions are multi-levelled and multi-faceted. The authors recommend that evaluations of self-efficacy should be conducted as part of the supervision process. They advocate the integration of training, supervision and service development models as an efficient and effective strategy.

Boast, N. & Chesterman, P. (1995) Black people and secure psychiatric facilities. *British Journal of Criminology*, **35**, 218–235.

Introduction

This literature review takes an in-depth look at a multiplicity of factors thought to be behind the over-representation of African–Caribbean people within secure psychiatric hospitals in the UK. This includes consideration of the characteristics of psychiatric patients, such as rates of illness or psychiatric morbidity, and those inherent to the system, such as stereotyping or institutional racism.

Review

There has been much criticism that courts and the police discriminate against Black people and some research has shown that Black people are more prone to arrest for violent crime, more likely to be charged immediately and less likely to be cautioned or referred to juvenile authorities. However, this evidence is confused by studies which have not found a bias, for example in relation to sentencing.

Another paradox pointed out by the reviewers is that, even though African–Caribbean patients are more frequently detained under the Mental Health Act, the overall rate of admission for the group corresponds to that for other migrant peoples.

Concepts of mental disorder (such as mental illness, behavioural disturbance, insight, risk to others), perceptions of personality and criminality, and availability of psychiatric services are all factors that have been shown to influence whether or not a patient is detained compulsorily. The writers investigate each of these factors but conclude that it is socio-economic disadvantage rather than systematic discrimination within the health and criminal justice systems that accounts for the over-representation of Black people in secure psychiatric facilities. They also point out that factors such as the lack of targeted community facilities, staff attitudes and Black people's antipathy to psychiatry all lead to delays in psychiatric presentation. These delays may in turn result in Black people presenting to services at times of personal crisis.

Bracken, P., Greenslade, L., Griffin, B. & Smyth, M. (1998) Mental health and ethnicity: an Irish dimension. *British Journal of Psychiatry,* **172**, 103–105.

In this editorial, the authors highlight issues of ethnicity, culture and racism in relation to the mental health of the Irish. Irish-born people make up 1.5% of the British population, and including Irish parentage increases the number to 4.6% of the total population. Using data from earlier studies, these authors point out that the rates of schizophrenia and other psychoses are nearly twice as high among the Irish compared with the indigenous population, whereas personality disorders are less likely, and the rate of alcoholism is nearly 10 times higher. Although these are admission data and admission rates are influenced by a number of factors, these are more likely to be related to social factors like poverty, unemployment and social isolation. The authors propose that the category 'White' requires substantial re-examination, and neglect of the Irish dimension must be overcome. The Irish are a colonised people and their needs must be understood and quantitative and qualitative research be taken seriously in this group.

Brown, I. & Hullin, R. (1992) A study of sentencing in the Leeds magistrates' courts. *British Journal of Criminology,* **32**, 41–53.

Introduction

Discrimination against Black people can be readily observed in UK courts. However, despite systematic research, explanations for this phenomenon are in short supply, mainly because of the contradictory nature of the research findings themselves. For example, while some classic studies have shown that the over-representation of Black people cannot be explained by bias in sentencing, others have suggested that there is racial discrimination in sentencing. These conflicting findings may partially be explained by errors in research design. The authors attempt to clarify the picture by carrying out a further study of sentencing practices.

Method

Unbeknown to magistrates at the time, information was collected about all defendants sentenced for trial in Leeds magistrates' and crown courts, over a nine-month period. Defendants who were not Leeds residents were excluded from the final sample. The data collected included basic demographic information and details of the most serious offence and of sentence. If the defendant had a previous criminal record, the number of previous convictions, the number of convictions for the same offence, information about their three most serious previous disposals for the same offence, the number of previous custodial sentences and the most severe previous sentence were collected.

The researchers aimed to test three hypotheses: first, that ethnic minority offenders would be more likely to receive custodial sentences; secondly, that ethnic minority offenders would be less likely to receive the full range of non-custodial sentences; and finally, that more ethnic minority offenders would be committed to crown court for trial by magistrates, and a greater proportion of them would elect for trial by jury.

Results

Over the test period, 90.7% of defendants were found to be White, 5.8% African–Caribbean, 3.2% Asian and 0.3% from other ethnic groups. Their corresponding proportions in the local population were 93.6%, 1.9%, 3.5% and 1.0%, respectively. The African–Caribbean group contained a higher proportion of women than the other ethnic groups, with Asians having the lowest. A significant proportion of African–Caribbeans of both genders were in the 21–25-year age range. Twice the proportion of White and Asian defendants were employed compared with African–Caribbean defendants. The range of offences with which African–Caribbean and Asian defendants were charged was significantly different from that with which White defendants were charged. African–Caribbeans tended to be charged with more violent offences, but with fewer involving dishonesty. However, these results varied across the age groups. African–Caribbean defendants under 21 were convicted of committing proportionally fewer violent offences.

Significantly more African–Caribbeans had a criminal record. There was no difference between the seriousness of previous convictions across ethnic groups. However, Asian defendants were significantly more likely to be first offenders.

Overall, the sentences given to defendants did not differ significantly across ethnic groups. However, African–Caribbeans in the 26–30-year age group were more likely to be given custodial sentences. Other factors, such as criminal record, were similar. When committals for sentence were added to the figures, the differences found disappeared. African–Caribbean women had a more serious history of convictions and were more likely to be given a custodial sentence than women from the other ethnic groups. Twice the proportion of African–Caribbean as of White defendants received a custodial sentence for theft. The only difference between the two groups was that African–Caribbeans' previous convictions for theft were likely to have been more recent. No differences were found between the groups in terms of non-custodial sentences.

More African–Caribbean than White defendants were committed for trial to the crown court by magistrates upon the recommendation of the Crown Prosecution Service. When crimes were considered separately, only in relation to drug offences was there a significant difference in the numbers committed by magistrates.

Discussion

The proportion of African–Caribbean and Asian people in Leeds is higher than their proportions nationally. However, the authors contend that it is unlikely that the sample is atypical. They do acknowledge, though, that generalisations may be difficult if court and police practices differ nationally. The definition of custodial sentence used in the study differs from that of other studies in that it includes suspended sentences and committals to crown court.

The researchers did not find any real evidence in support of their first hypothesis that African–Caribbeans receive more custodial sentences. The only real area of difference was in the number of African–Caribbeans committed to crown court for trial. Further research, they say, is needed to investigate whether this difference is affected by the circumstances in which the crime was committed.

African–Caribbeans are over-represented in the sample compared with their proportion in the local population and the results suggest that they are offending at a younger age than Whites. This is another area that needs further study.

Although African–Caribbeans were more likely to be unemployed they were not less likely to be fined. In the case of crimes against the person, especially where no injury was sustained, a combination of a higher reporting rate among White victims and failure on behalf of the courts to downgrade these offences may explain why more African–Carbbeans are charged with these crimes; but this still leaves the question of why fewer African–Caribbeans under 21 years are charged with violent offences.

Burnett, R., Mallett, R., Bhugra, D., Hutchinson, G. and Leff, J. (1999) The first contact of patients with schizophrenia with psychiatric services: social factors and pathways to care in a multi-ethnic population. *Psychological Medicine*, **29**, 475–483.

Introduction

For first contact of patients with schizophrenia, pathways into care are determined by a number of factors including accessibility to services, severity of symptoms, ethnicity, social factors and absence of contact with primary care. Studies have shown mixed findings so far.

Method

Over a two-year period in two catchment areas in London, first contact cases of schizophrenia were identified. Pathways into care were obtained using personal and psychiatric history schedules, which were identified by relatives or patients themselves.

Results

The final sample of 100 included 38 Whites, 38 African–Caribbeans and 24 Asians. Fewer people in the African–Caribbean group went via their general practitioner (GP). A quarter of African–Caribbeans had police involved in their pathway, compared with 16% Whites and 4% Asians. These patients were more likely to be unemployed and those who came through prison were more likely to live alone. African–Caribbeans were least likely to be referred by their GPs, but those who followed this pathway were more likely to have reached vocational or tertiary education. In total, 28% of patients were admitted to hospital under section but ethnic status had no effect on the likelihood of compulsory admission. Not surprisingly, those who were referred through their GPs were less likely to be detained compulsorily.

African–Caribbeans who lived alone were more likely to be sectioned than African–Caribbeans who lived with friends or family.

These findings confirm pervious findings that ethnic status is not a key factor in pathways to care or rates of compulsory admission for the initial contact of patients with psychiatric services. Social isolation and unemployment along with low educational status all contribute to compulsory admission. The role of the GP as gatekeeper becomes extremely important. The differences between the minority ethnic groups are linked with socio-demographic characteristics such as age, living with family and being unemployed. Strong social and family networks among Asians may well delay their presentation and pathway though their GP.

Discussion

The number of Asian patients included, although the largest reported in a study so far, is still low. The two catchment areas were perhaps not entirely representative of the UK population as a whole. The study also reports findings from the Camberwell case register which confirms that rates of compulsory admission in first contact do not differ between African–Caribbeans and Whites, but that although readmission rates are lower for African–Caribbeans, the rates of compulsory admission are disproportionately higher.

Button, E., Reveley, C. & Palmer, R. (1998) An ethnic comparison of eating attitudes and associated problems in young British women. *International Journal of Eating Disorders*, **23**, 317–323.

Introeduction

Although rates of eating disorders may vary in British Asian groups, certain family characteristics have been linked with these rates. These include maternal control and social factors like gender roles. The authors set out to examine rates of eating problems in different ethnic groups and their correlation with anxiety, depression and self-esteem.

Method

A target of 486 women aged 18–27 were identified from general practice surgery registers and approached by post. The questionnaire included demographic details, weight and eating, EAT–26, the

Hospital Anxiety and Depression scale and three vignettes to determine help-seeking behaviour. The vignettes covered headache, depression and eating behaviour.

Results

Of 486 approached, 15 had moved or were ineligible. Of the remaining people, 235 responded (49.9%). Ethnic groups were categorised as Caucasian (60%), Asian (26%), Black (11%) and other (3%). Asians were less likely to be single, living away from parents or partner or working. There were no significant ethnic differences on weight perception, exercise or using methods such as diuretics or laxatives. Caucasians were more likely to use vomiting. There were no differences in health-seeking behaviour or anxiety and depression.

These findings suggest that no generalisations can be made according to ethnic differences.

Discussion

The overall response rates although low are acceptable. A significant number of Asians were Sikh, which does not reflect the local population composition.

Callan, A. (1996) Schizophrenia in Afro-Caribbean immigrants. *Journal of the Royal Society of Medicine*, **89**, 253–256.

Introduction

Research on schizophrenia and the African–Caribbean community in the UK has tended to concentrate on incidence and prevalence rates and on the accuracy of diagnosis. This study attempts to discover, first, whether formal admission rates are higher for African–Caribbeans when differences in age, gender and diagnoses are taken into account; and secondly, whether a diagnosis of schizophrenia has the same outcome for African–Caribbeans as for White patients.

Method

Included in the study were patients born in the West Indies admitted, with a diagnosis of schizophrenia, between 1975 and 1982 to an 800-

bed mental hospital serving four London boroughs. The control group comprised White British patients matched in terms of year of admission, gender and age (within five years). Patients over 45, those whose illness had lasted for longer than five years, non-African–Caribbean West Indians and British-born non-Whites were excluded from the study. Demographic information, family history of mental illness, number of admissions, length of stay, duration of illness before admission and referrer were all extracted from hospital records. The amount of medication patients received during their admission was also recorded. Research and diagnostic criteria to determine diagnosis were applied to patient records.

Results

Fifty African–Caribbean patients and 94 White British patients were admitted with a diagnosis of schizophrenia during the period under investigation. The 24 African–Caribbean men in the sample were matched with 24 White British men but the 26 African–Caribbean women could be matched with only 17 White British women. Among those for whom the information was available, 34% of African–Caribbean patients and 67% of White British patients had a family history of mental illness. Approximately half of the patients in both ethnic groups were given a diagnosis (according to Research Diagnostic Criteria) of schizophrenia, while approximately 20% met the criteria for atypical psychosis, and 16% of African–Caribbean and 24% of White British patients met the criteria for a depressive disorder not otherwise specified. White British patients tended to have more negative symptoms but this difference was not significant. Similarities were found between the two ethnic groups in terms of average number of readmissions and length of time between index admission and a patient's last contact with services. Twenty African–Caribbean and eight White British patients had only one admission. The duration of readmissions was nearly twice as long for White British patients as a whole, but the difference between the ethnic groups was larger for women. There were no differences in terms of mode of onset of the illness, but 63% of African–Caribbean compared with only 30% of White patients had been ill for less than one week on admission. African–Caribbean patients experienced an excess of police referrals at the expense of referrals from general practitioners. African–Caribbean men and women had higher rates of formal admissions than their White counterparts. No differences were found in the proportions of patients discharged on depot medication or in the dosage of depot or oral medication. However, while in-patients, White British men received significantly higher doses of medication.

Discussion

African–Caribbean and White patients had similar diagnostic profiles. The results indicate that the increased rates of schizophrenia reported in African–Caribbean patients represents a real difference between the ethnic groups – although it seems that the illness is more benign in African–Caribbeans. The findings also confirmed that the higher rates of compulsory detention reported remain when gender, age and diagnosis are taken into account. The author suggests that the results might have been due to differences in the way patients interact with services at several levels. Differences in the use of specialist services, in the presentation of illness and bias in health professionals' perception of Black patients are all seen as possible reasons for the discrepancies found. The author suggests that the higher rates of police involvement in African–Caribbean referrals are probably a consequence of the patient's family initiating contact with the police, rather than of police racism.

Callan, A. & Littlewood, R. (1998) Patient satisfaction: ethnic origin or explanatory model? *International Journal of Social Psychiatry*, **44**, 1–11.

Introduction

Assessment of patient satisfaction has emerged from a series of divergent ideological concerns such as compliance, the introduction of market economy and growth of users' movements. These have all contributed to an upsurge in measuring patient satisfaction with psychiatric services in a number of settings. The authors propose that where patients' and professionals' explanatory models merge, satisfaction is likely to be higher.

Method

An open-ended questionnaire consisting of 58 questions was developed with responses on a Likert scale. Explanatory models were explored using Kleinman's questions. All Black and ethnic minority patients admitted to a hospital in London over a nine-month period were interviewed. The control patients were consecutive White patients admitted to the same unit over a six-week period. Socio-demographic details and ethnicity were noted and patients interviewed once dates for discharge had been set.

Results

Ninety-six Black and ethnic minority patients and 29 Whites were eligible to take part in the study. Only 62 Black and ethnic minority patients and 19 White patients were interviewed. Six patients from the former group refused to take part, 9 were AWOL and 18 were either too ill or had precipitor discharge compared with nil, 2 and 6 from the latter group. Gender and age distribution across the two groups were broadly similar but Blacks were more likely to have had psychoses, longer duration, involuntary admission and no fixed address.

There were no significant differences in overall satisfaction between the ethnic groups, but three items which did show significant differences were Blacks being allowed off the ward, lower satisfaction among Whites with ward rounds, and help provided to deal with problems more effectively. Convergent explanatory models were more likely to be satisfied even when Mental Health Act status was taken into account.

The minority patients are able to express their satisfaction with services and do not feel that they are being given substandard care. The conundrum of high rates of psychoses and Mental Health Act detention has not been solved yet. The use of explanatory models deserves to be studied further in future studies.

Discussion

Attrition rates are very high and it is likely that those who were AWOL or refused were voting with their feet by virtue of higher levels of dissatisfaction. The measurement of explanatory models is relatively crude; it would have been more useful to ask the staff about their perceptions. The significant relationship between explanatory model type and questions on patient autonomy need to be studied further.

Castle, D., Wessely, S., Der, G. & Murray, R. M. (1991) The incidence of operationally defined schizophrenia in Camberwell, 1965–1984. *British Journal of Psychiatry*, **159**, 790–794.

Introduction

Research carried out in various parts of the world, from Scotland to Australia, has concluded that the incidence of schizophrenia has fallen over the past 30 years or more. The authors were therefore surprised to observe that a register recording the first contacts of all psychiatric patients in Camberwell did not show a concomitant decrease, and set out to investigate this anomaly.

Method

The researchers obtained a list of all patients who experienced their first contact with psychiatric services between 1965 and 1984, who were resident in Camberwell, south London, and who had been given a diagnosis of schizophrenic psychosis (meeting ICD–9 criteria) – excluding those whose illness clearly had an organic basis and those who had previously received treatment elsewhere. Valid cases totalled 486. Each patient's case notes were analysed and the demographic characteristics were recorded. The researchers also applied the Operational Checklist for Psychotic Illness, which covers a range of operational definitions – ICD–9, DSM–III and Research Diagnostic Criteria (RDC) – for schizophrenia, to each case. Information regarding the general population of Camberwell was obtained from census data.

Results

The study period was divided into four time cohorts and the incidence rates of schizophrenia were calculated for each. Using all three definitions, the rate of schizophrenia was found to have risen in the total period under study. In order to discover what effect the ethnicity of the sample may be exerting on these results, the researchers ascertained the percentages of both Caribbean-born and British-born African–Caribbeans among the total number of patients who fulfilled the RDC definition of schizophrenia, and found that in each time cohort their numbers far exceeded those of all individuals born in Britain.

Discussion

The authors discuss the reasons why they should have obtained findings which so sharply contrast those of other researchers. They consider whether their method may have been flawed, but suggest that using standardised criteria for schizophrenia should have excluded any bias arising from changing diagnostic practices. They state that the case notes examined were thorough. It is suggested that these findings are more likely to result from changes to the population of Camberwell, most importantly the increase in the proportion of African–Caribbeans; census returns showed that the proportion of those born in the West Indies and living in Camberwell rose from 2.5% in 1961 to 6.6% in 1981. Since a number of studies have shown that rates of schizophrenia among African–Caribbeans compared with Whites are 3–6 times higher for those born abroad and 7–14 times higher for those born in Britain, it seems likely that this change is responsible for at least part of the difference.

Cochrane, R. & Howell, M. (1995) Drinking patterns of black and white men in the West Midlands. *Social Psychiatry and Psychiatric Epidemiology*, **30**, 139–156.

Introduction

This study took place against a background of existing research which suggests that people of African–Caribbean origin living in the UK suffer from fewer alcohol-related problems than their White counterparts. This study aimed to discover whether the pattern of alcohol use differed between African–Caribbean and White men in the West Midlands, whether the African–Caribbean men *did* suffer fewer alcohol-related problems, and whether the effect was the same for those born in the Caribbean as for those born in Britain.

Method

The researchers interviewed a random sample of 200 Black men (drawn from the lists of six general practice surgeries in Birmingham) and collected demographic information, information about drinking patterns, including how often the respondent had an alcoholic drink and whether he had ever sought or received treatment for an alcohol-related problem, and information about psychological well-being. The data were compared with data obtained from a group of 170 White males, gathered during the course of an earlier study.

Results

The White men were more evenly distributed through the age categories, but more Black men were aged over 50. Higher proportions of the White men were married and employed. The Black men were found to be over-represented in the lower social classes and under-represented in the top social classes.

For both Black and White men, beer was the most frequently consumed drink, and most drinking took place at weekends. Twenty per cent of Black men abstained from drinking, in comparison with 4.7% of Whites. Among the White men, 35.5% drank more than three times a week, comapred with 16.5% of Black men. Only 8% of Black men reported drinking more than 20 units in the week before the interview, as opposed to 22% of the White men. No Black men reported getting drunk every week, whereas 6.5% of White men admitted that they did. White men appeared much more likely to have become involved in a fight or to have come to the attention to the police in connection with their drinking. No Black men had sought treatment for an alcohol-related problem, but 3.5% of White men had done so. Differences in drinking habits were not found to be attributable to any differences in demographic characteristics of the two groups, and there were very few differences found between the Black men born in the UK and those born in the Caribbean.

Discussion

The pattern of consumption among the Black and White samples was found to be virtually the same, but frequency and consumption were very different. The researchers concluded that Black men in England drink much less alcohol than do White men, and suggest that this may be due to their greater likelihood of being a member of the Pentecostal Church, which adopts a strict attitude towards drinking.

Cole, E., Leavey, G., King, M., Johnson-Sabine, E. & Hoar, A. (1995) Pathways to care for patients with a first episode of psychosis – a comparison of ethnic groups. *British Journal of Psychiatry*, **167**, 770–776.

Introduction

A number of studies have reported that Black and ethnic minority patients in their pathway to psychiatric care are less likely to be involved with a general practitioner, and are more likely to come into contact with mental health services through police, civil or court compulsory admissions. The result is that the pathway taken to reach care is likely to be of a less desirable nature. However, existing research has tended not to distinguish between patients with a first onset of psychosis and those with a chronic illness. This study focused on those experiencing their first onset of psychotic illness (because first experiences of services may affect future engagement) and examined the effect of ethnicity on the pathway taken to reach care.

Method

One hospital's catchment area was screened for a year to detect all new cases of psychotic illness. All patients were interviewed to obtain information regarding their demographic characteristics, ethnicity, psychiatric history, current mental state, mode of onset of their illness, and pathway to care. Information was corroborated by a key informant, and further information was taken from case files where necessary.

Results

Ninety-three patients, mean age 29 years, were recruited to the study. Eighty-five per cent had been born abroad or had one parent born abroad. Seventy-five per cent were unemployed. The majority had initially consulted a health or social service agency, and there was no difference between the different ethnic groups in this regard. For all patients, a general practitioner was most commonly consulted first. Patients who lived alone were found to be most likely to consult a non-medical agency first. Black patients were most likely to be compulsorily admitted, but this was not statistically significant. The absence of a family or friend to aid help-seeking was found to predict compulsory admission and admission under Section 136 of the Mental Health Act. Eighteen per cent of the patients sought advice from a religious agency, but there were no significant variations between the ethnic groups. The majority of patients came into contact with services one month or more after the first symptoms of their illness. Black patients were slightly more likely to present later, but this was not statistically significant – only the fact of being single predicted a later presentation. Diagnostic categories were divided into 'schizophrenia certain to possible' and 'no schizophrenia'. The researchers did not find significant differences between the two diagnostic groups in terms of any of the variables under study.

Discussion

Patient ethnicity was not found significantly to determine the pathway taken by these patients experiencing their first onset of psychosis. The fact of the patient being able to negotiate help or to have help arranged by relatives and friends seemed much more significant factors in the patient taking a desirable pathway. The researchers therefore suggest that patients who do not have social support should receive more attention, and that support should be given to friends and relatives who are providing help for sick relatives.

Collins, D., Dimsdale, J. E. & Wilkins, D. (1992) Consultation/ liaison psychiatry utilization patterns in different cultural groups. *Psychosomatic Medicine*, **54**, 240–245.

Introduction

Ethnicity has been shown to have an impact on psychiatric diagnosis and treatment. The need to understand cross-cultural issues in a consultation setting is felt, by the authors, to be of increasing importance because of ongoing increases in the ethnic diversity of patients in US general hospitals. This study investigated ethnic patterns in the psychiatric referrals of patients in a general hospital.

Method

The study took place in a 400-bed general teaching hospital. Details of the 504 psychiatric consultations carried out between July 1989 and April 1990 were examined. Patients' ethnic origins, the reasons for referral and the types of psychiatric problems found were investigated.

Results

The ethnicity of 476 of the 504 patients given psychiatric referrals was noted in hospital records. A significant difference was found in the proportions that the patients referred for psychiatric consultation represented of all referrals of patients of their ethnic group to the general hospital (1.5% of Hispanic patients, 4.3% of White patients, 4.2% of Black patients and 3.1% of Asian patients). Ethnicity was also found to be associated with the reason for consultations. Hispanic patients tended to be referred for evaluation of depression/ suicidal behaviour. They more frequently received a diagnosis of adjustment disorder than other ethnic groups and less frequently one of substance misuse. They were no more likely to receive a diagnosis of affective disorder. Black patients were more likely than other ethnic groups to be referred for evaluation of grossly abnormal mental status. Substance misuse was seen as the most common cause for this behaviour, followed by affective disorders, adjustment disorders and personality disorders. Black patients were more likely to receive a diagnosis of thought disorder and delirium compared with other ethnic groups. White patients were more likely to be diagnosed with dementia.

Discussion

The researchers find it difficult to explain the lower rate of referral of Hispanics, especially as this group did not seem to be any more resistant to psychiatric referral. Despite being less likely to be referred for depression or suicidal behaviour, Black patients were just as likely as other ethnic groups to receive a diagnosis of affective disorder. This supports other research that has found that affective disorders in Black people are not being recognised in primary care.

The increased frequency with which Black patients were being referred for assessment of abnormal mental status was in line with the increased likelihood of a primary diagnosis of thought disorder or delirium. Although reasons for this discrepancy are unclear, White patients, who were more likely to be diagnosed with dementia, tended to be older than patients from other ethnic groups. The rate of substance misuse was found to vary with ethnicity; for example, Hispanics were less likely to have this diagnosis, contrary to the findings of other studies. The reasons for this finding are also unclear. Further study is needed to investigate the results observed. The authors suggest that comparisons across socio-economic groups may also prove valuable.

Copeland, J. R. M. (1968) Aspects of mental illness in West African students. *Social Psychiatry*, **3**, 7–13.

Introduction

Researchers have reported high levels of schizophrenic illness in immigrants in different parts of the world. West African students in the UK, as temporary immigrants, experience many of the difficulties of permanent immigrants. Researchers have postulated that there is a connection between the schizoid character and emigration. One would expect West African students, who usually intend to return home, to have less of any predispositional personality factors associated with migration. Research has also shown that cultural factors affect the expression of mental illness in Africans.

Method

Sixty students of West African origin admitted to three hospitals in south London with severe mental illness were included in the study. All had fallen ill either during their course of study or just before starting it. Data were collected from hospital case notes. Patients were followed up by contacting a variety of sources, such as hospitals that had requested patient discharge summaries, general practitioners, the students' colleges, relatives (both in Britain and abroad) and, in some cases, patients themselves.

Results

There were 52 men and 8 women, of whom 33 were given a diagnosis of schizophrenia, 8 of schizoaffective psychosis, 2 of mania, 11 of depression, 3 of mixed affective disorder and 3 of a paranoid state. Sixty per cent of the students were admitted through acute emergency wards. Fifteen were seen during their first admission by a psychiatrically trained doctor or nurse from their county of origin. These doctors and nurses always agreed with the diagnoses given.

The length of psychiatric follow-up varied from six months to six years, but over half were followed up for at least three years. The students diagnosed with schizophrenia relapsed more frequently than others. Half of the 26 students diagnosed with schizophrenia refused to accept the recommendation of repatriation. Three of the four students who returned after repatriation relapsed within weeks. Twenty-one patients in total were repatriated, mostly between one and eight years after the first episode of psychiatric illness.

Thirty-one students were either repatriated or abandoned their course of study without taking further examinations, while six students tried but failed to pass them. Eight passed further examinations but eventually failed to qualify. Five students both passed and qualified. The further academic achievements of 10 of the students was not known.

Discussion

Most initial diagnoses were confirmed on subsequent admissions. Fifty-seven of the 60 students admitted were found to have persecutory symptoms. This included the depressed students. However, the researcher does not feel that this finding provides a reason why low levels of depression are recorded in Africans. The suggestion is that in this group, persecutory ideas are culturally derived from superstitions and the existence of polygamy. It is felt that removing persecutory symptoms from consideration helps to provide an accurate diagnosis. Relatives of West African patients when present during consultations tended to agree with the patient's declarations of being poisoned. However, relatives also tended to agree that the patient was mentally ill because of what was seen as odd behaviour, such as the open accusation of 'persecutors'.

Overall, the academic achievements of students after their first admission was poor. A diagnosis of schizophrenia and more than one admission were most highly associated with academic failure.

Previous research has shown that students who are repatriated respond better to treatment – although the relapse rate was still found to be high. Not enough of those repatriated could be followed up to allow the researcher to draw any clear conclusion.

Davies, S., Thornicroft, G., Leese, M., Higginbotham, A. & Phelan, M. (1996) Ethnic differences in risk of compulsory psychiatric admission among representative cases of psychosis in London. *British Medical Journal,* **312,** 533–537.

Introduction

Previous research had reported higher rates of severe mental illness and higher rates of admission to hospital within the African–Caribbean population in the UK. This research aimed to examine rates of admission among those who had suffered a psychotic episode, and to discover whether rates of admission were higher in this group, independent of diagnosis.

Method

Researchers used a range of hospital and community sources to identify the period prevalence of psychotic disorders within two catchment areas in south London, in 1991. Standardised criteria were used to identify diagnosis and detention under the Mental Health Act was noted. The ethnic group of the individual was established using census classifications. Any person who had ever been diagnosed as suffering from a psychotic disorder was included. When a case was identified, additional data pertaining to socio-demographic characteristics, past diagnoses, all contacts with mental health services, contacts with police and details of compulsory admissions were also collected.

Results

ICD–10 diagnoses of psychotic disorder were identified in 439 cases (44.5% of these were, or had been, of schizophrenia). Ethnic group was established in 93.1% of cases. Most of the subjects were single, lived alone and were unemployed. There were no significant differences in the socio-demographic characteristics of the different ethnic groups, with the exception that Black patients tended to be younger.

Of the total sample, 51.1% had been sectioned under the Mental Health Act at some point in their lives, but the rate was significantly higher among Black patients than White patients. The mean number of admissions to hospital was significantly higher among the Black African and Black Caribbean groups than within the White group. The rates of detention under sections 2, 3 and 136 were significantly higher among the Black patients, and this was particularly prominent for section 136. An analysis of the risk of having been in contact with forensic mental health services showed that Black patients were, again, significantly more likely to have used these services.

Discussion

Rates of sectioning in South London were found to be higher overall than average rates for the UK, identified some years previously. However, reductions in the number of beds nationally may account for this discrepancy.

Both Black Africans and Black Caribbeans were more likely to have been compulsorily detained, and this was independent of diagnosis; they were also more likely to have been admitted to psychiatric intensive-care units or prisons. Black patients were younger than the White cohort, and therefore could not be said simply to have had a longer 'exposure time'.

Flannigan, C. B., Glover, G. R., Wing, J. K., Lewis, S. W., Bebbington, P. E. & Feeney, S. T. (1994) Inner London collaborative audit of admission in two health districts III: reasons for acute admission to psychiatric wards. *British Journal of Psychiatry*, **165**, 750–759.

Introduction

This paper is the third of a series reporting an audit of acute patients admitted to psychiatric wards in Hammersmith and Fulham and south Southwark. The paper is primarily concerned with the reasons for which patients were admitted. The previous papers had noted that in Southwark, rates for admission, bed use and period prevalence of admission were around 30% higher than in Hammersmith and Fulham, and that this appeared to be largely due to higher rates of admission for affective disorders in this borough.

Method

A sample of 266 patients was chosen. Details of the sampling procedure are described in the previous two papers. Patients' key workers were asked to provide details of the circumstances of the assessment, prodromal symptoms, frequency of contact with services before admission and clinical state. Clinical judgements were made as to whether the reasons given were major or contributory to the decision to admit the patient, and whether admission could have been prevented.

Results

Nearly all patients were found to be suffering from a major mental illness. Relief for the patient or carer, risk of self-harm and problems with medication were found to be the most common reasons for admission. At least one major reason, other than simply observation, was recorded for 224 out of the 226 patients. More patients with schizophrenia (as opposed to affective disorder) were admitted for observation only. Of the total sample, 19% were admitted to restart medication. There was a significant correlation between problems with medication and ethnicity (17% of White people versus 31% of African–Caribbeans). Almost one-third of the total sample had not experienced regular contact with specialist services or with their families before admission, but 40% were in contact with their general practitioners. Around two-thirds of all cases had exhibited prodromal symptoms before admission. Appropriate action was deemed not to have been taken in 10–15% of these cases. Approximately one-third of patients and two-thirds of carers had no straightforward way of requesting help.

Discussion

The two areas under study were both urban, of similar size and achieving similar scores on scales of deprivation. Bed use was 30% higher in Southwark as a result of higher admission rates for people with affective disorders. The most striking difference between the two boroughs, in terms of reasons for admission, was 'patient request and relief for carers' – which was almost unheard of as a reason for admission in Hammersmith and Fulham. 'Prevention of suicide' as a reason for admission was employed twice as frequently in Southwark. The researchers suggested that this may have a measurable effect on completed suicide rates in Hammersmith and Fulham.

Glover, G. R., Flannigan, C. B., Feeney, S. T., Wing, J. K., Bebbington, P. E. & Lewis, S. W. (1994) Admission of British Caribbeans to mental hospitals: is it a cohort effect? *Social Psychiatry and Psychiatric Epidemiology*, **29**, 282–284.

Introduction

Early research in the UK investigating the relationship between ethnicity and schizophrenia indicated that there were higher prevalence rates among Caribbean men than among members of other ethnic groups. The differences found in early studies were much smaller than those found in more recent research. Further investigations indicated that the differences found might be due to a cohort effect limited to members of the Caribbean community born after 1950. Researchers speculated first that the increased rates were a direct consequence of migration. Second, the possibility was also raised that the higher prevalence rates were due to exposure of Caribbean men to some infective agent in mid-foetal life to which women, resident in the UK, were usually immune. The authors speculate that if the second supposition were correct, the high rates of schizophrenia should be confined to men born before 1966, by which time migration from the Caribbean had all but stopped. The majority of Caribbean-born women resident in the UK should have had time to develop an immunity; thus children born to them in the late 1960s should not have been exposed to the infective agent. The researchers attempt to test this hypothesis.

Method

Demographic and outcome data were collected from a study of admissions in three London health districts for schizophrenia. Corresponding population data of the relevant catchment areas were collected using census figures.

Results

In the year 1976/77, British Caribbean men aged 15–24 and 25–34 years were most at risk of developing schizophrenia. By 1991, this increased risk had shifted to Caribbean men aged 25–34 and 35–44 years. In 1991, there were significantly fewer admissions of Caribbean men in the 15–24-year age range, and significantly more in the 35–44-year age range, than would have been expected from the 1984/85 distribution. Overall, the 1991 profile of incidence rates diverged significantly form the 1984/85 profile. There were much smaller variations in incidence rates for women and these did not reach significance. The age profiles of ethnic Whites of both genders with schizophrenia showed no significant shift.

Discussion

The above findings could indicate the tail end of an epidemic. However, there is a need to be cautious when interpreting these findings because the results could have been skewed by:

(a) the relatively small numbers of admissions in some age and gender groups;
(b) the inclusion of multiple admissions of individual patients;
(c) the variety of methods used for classifying ethnicity across different time periods;
(d) data for different years being drawn from patients living in different areas of London;
(e) underestimation of the numbers of Caribbeans in the general population, particularly where the 1991 census data were used to calculate incidence rates.

There is an urgent need for more extensive work to be done in this area.

Goddard, N., Subotsky, F. & Fombonne, E. (1996) Ethnicity and adolescent deliberate self-harm. *Journal of Adolescence*, **19**, 513–521.

Introduction

The 1994 Health Advisory Service's *Thematic Review of Suicide Prevention* draws particular attention to the problem of suicide behaviour in children and adolescents. However, the actual level of deliberate self-harm (DSH) among adolescents is difficult to quantify because no comprehensive statistics exist. The studies that have attempted to quantify the problem have been hampered by differences in the definitions of DSH and the age groupings used in data collection. Research has shown, however, that there are specific factors associated with DSH – for example, a third of adolescents who present after an overdose live in single-parent families. The issue of ethnicity as a factor in adolescent DSH has not received much attention. One recent UK study found no differences in the rates of DSH among the Asian and White populations, although Asians had higher rates of depression and hopelessness, were more socially isolated and had longer periods of premeditation. Other studies have suggested that lower rates of DSH exist in the Black population. The aim of this study was to compare DSH referral rates by ethnicity and to investigate differences between the Black and White adolescents referred.

Method

The case notes of all referrals made, between January 1990 and December 1992, to the department of child and adolescent psychiatry of a south London hospital were reviewed. Children over 10 years who were referred for their first episode of DSH were included in the study. There were 100 cases. Demographic information and details of variables important to DSH, such as the method used and the presence of substance misuse, were collected. In addition, an item sheet with details of symptoms, diagnosis, psychosocial facts and treatment was filled in for all patients. The ethnicity of subjects was classified according to the 1991 census and local population data were calculated using the same census information. If 40% or more of the data required for analysis were missing, patients were excluded from the study.

Results

The ethnicity of the cases identified as appropriate for analysis was 64 White, 20 Black Caribbean, 2 Black African, 6 Black other, 2 Asian and 6 other (including mixed race). For subsequent analysis, the sample was divided into three broader groups of White, Black and other. The number of cases identified in each group reflected their proportions in the local community; however, the predominance of females in the Black and White groups was found to be significant. There were no significant differences found between the Black and White groups in terms of the sociodemographic factors investigated. In terms of DSH characteristics, both groups had high rates of family break-up but White adolescents were twice as likely to have a family psychiatric history. This difference did not quite reach significance. Patients in the Black and White groups did not differ significantly on any of the other background characteristics of DSH. Only in relation to two of the psychosocial stressors investigated (persecution/discrimination and migration/social transplantation) was there a significant difference between the two groups – for Black male adolescents, these two stressors were more common. Ethnicity was not found to affect outcome or treatment.

Discussion

The authors begin by discussing some of the methodological problems associated with the study, such as referral bias. The fact that only DSH cases in the form of self-poisoning were identified may, they say, point to another source of bias. Despite reported under-utilisation of services by ethnic minority adolescents, the research found referral rates among all communities to be similar to their proportions in the wider population. Overall, the two groups showed few differences, contrary to the findings of previous studies.

The one difference found between the groups leads the authors to suggest that social stressors may be a significant factor in DSH in Black male adolescents and they recommend further research is carried out in this area.

Gupta, S. (1991) Psychosis in migrants from the Indian subcontinent and English-born controls – a preliminary study on the use of psychiatric services. *British Journal of Psychiatry*, **159**, 222–225.

Introduction

A large number of existing research studies had shown that among immigrants to the UK (including those from the Indian subcontinent), rates of diagnosis of schizophrenia are significantly higher than rates found in the indigenous population. This study aimed to compare the subsequent involvement with psychiatric services of a group of Asian immigrants with a diagnosis of non-organic adult psychosis with that of a matched group of English-born controls.

Method

The author obtained a sample of 86 first-generation Asian immigrants born on the Indian subcontinent who were seen at the Bethlem and Maudsley hospitals (London) between 1969 and 1983 and who had been given a diagnosis of functional psychosis. They were compared with a sample of patients who were seen at the hospitals during the same time period, and who were matched by date of admission and age, but who had been born in England. Case notes were studied and the two groups compared in terms of the total length of time spent as an in-patient, the total number of separate in-patient admissions in a year, and the average duration of each in-patient stay, two and five years after their initial contact with services, and up to the date that the case notes were being analysed.

Results

A greater proportion of the Asian sample was male (67% in comparison with 43% of the controls). More of the Asian sample were married or cohabiting. Approximately two-thirds of the Asian group had spent less than 1% of the total follow-up time in hospital, in comparison with only half of the controls. Asian patients had had fewer in-patient episodes at the two- and five-year follow-up, and the in-patient episodes which did occur were significantly shorter on average than those of the controls.

Discussion

The author discusses possible explanations for these findings, and acknowledges that one could be bias. It is pointed out that it may be that Asian patients were more mobile than control patients, and were perhaps readmitted to other hospitals. However, when the notes were first examined, it was found that similar proportions of patients in the two groups were found still to be registered with the same general practitioner they had on first contact, which may suggest that this is not the case. The author goes on to suggest that sociocultural factors may be responsible for the differentials observed, and points out that attending a psychiatric hospital in India carries a profound stigma. It is also suggested that Asian patients may have extended social networks (indeed, more Asian subjects in the study were found to be living with a partner at the time of first contact) and that this could have enabled them to avoid readmission. Gupta also suggests that there may be constitutional differences in the two samples and calls for this possibility to be researched.

Harrison, G., Cooper, J. E. & Gancarczyk, R. (1991) Changes in the administrative incidence of schizophrenia. *British Journal of Psychiatry*, **159**, 811–816.

Introduction

Some studies had suggested that first-admission rates for schizophrenia had declined by over 50% and that schizophrenia was a 'disappearing disorder'. The researchers point out problems in making such conclusions from data based on admission rates because changes in the different responses/interventions that general practitioners have used over time could affect admission rates – increased use of neuroleptics by general practitioners may prevent full onset and need for admission. New diagnostic criteria brought about by the introduction of DSM–III in 1980 may also have had an effect. The researchers suggest that despite the possibility of 'diagnostic drift', psychiatric case registers provide the most stable data, over time, when measuring 'administrative' incidence. This study used data from the Nottingham psychiatric case register in an effort to determine whether the administrative incidence of schizophrenia in the area had in fact fallen.

Method

Included in the Nottingham case register were details of all psychiatric contacts between 1975 and 1987 within Mapperly Hospital's catchment area. The methods of establishing diagnoses had undergone little change in the period, as the ICD–8 and ICD–9 criteria used in the respective years for schizophrenia and related disorders were similar. Information about first contacts under a range of diagnoses was collated along with information from the 1981 census. The 'administrative' incidence of schizophrenia over time was determined using linear regression.

Results

The study highlighted an increasing trend not to admit patients with a first-contact diagnosis of schizophrenia. No significant decrease in first-contact rates overall was found. However, a significant increase in the rates of paranoid states and reactive psychosis was identified. The difference in ICD–8 and ICD–9 diagnostic tools were thought to account for the drop in figures for affective psychosis, as evidence showed that under ICD–9 the condition was recorded as a 'depressive condition not elsewhere classified'.

Discussion

The authors point out that if hospital admission rates had been used as a measure of the incidence of schizophrenia, a decline would have been reported. However, including patients not admitted and using a broad definition of schizophrenia, an increase in incidence was found. They note that studies in both Oxford and Aberdeen also using first-contact information as a whole did in fact report falling rates. The researchers ask why their results differed. They do not feel that the diagnostic criteria they used were responsible. They point out that changes in community mental health provision – sectorisation, multi-disciplinary working and more effective liaison with general practitioners – make it less likely that people with schizophrenia living in the community are missed. They feel that changes in the local population may also have been a factor – research has reported higher rates of schizophrenia in African–Caribbean migrants and the area has considerably more African–Caribbeans than either Oxford or Aberdeen.

Harrison, G., Glazebrook, C., Brewin, J., Cantwell, R., Dalkin, T., Fox, R., Jones, P. & Medley, I. (1997) Increased incidence of psychotic disorders in migrants from the Caribbean to the United Kingdom. *Psychological Medicine*, **27**, 799–806.

Introduction

Despite the methodological problems that have characterised much of the work to investigate the relationship between migration and the incidence of psychotic disorders, the finding that African–Caribbeans are at increased risk of schizophrenia and related psychoses has proved remarkably robust. This paper reports on the result of research carried out in Nottingham to test the hypothesis that no difference in incidence rates exist. The assumption is that previous findings occurred because of bias in acquiring and defining appropriate cases or because of errors that arose from incorrect estimation of the numbers of African–Caribbeans in the local population.

Method

The researchers estimated the size of the population at risk by adjusting the 1991 census data as recommended by the Office of Population Censuses and Survey's guidelines, to adjust for the under-counting of African–Caribbean and 'Black other' males in the census figures. The researchers added the data for these groups together because, unlike in other parts of the UK, it could safely be assumed that most in the 'Black other' category were, in fact, of African–Caribbean origin. The figures for the local African–Caribbean male population were increased further until their numbers were equal to those reported for Black females in the area. Thus the official 1991 census estimate for African–Caribbean men overall was increased by 10% and in the case of men in the 20–29-year age range by 30%.

All potential access points to local psychiatric services were surveyed regularly and every patient with a potential diagnosis of psychosis, in contact with services for the first time, was interviewed. A patient's personal and family histories were obtained by direct interview or, if the patient refused this, from case notes. Assessments were carried out using a number of instruments and for each case a diagnostic meeting was held to explore other sources of information.

Results

The researchers found 124 patients of European origin and 32 of African–Caribbean origin who met the inclusion criteria. Incidence rates were calculated, for both psychoses generally and schizophrenia specifically, for a range of different age groups. Rates of psychoses for African–Caribbeans in the different age groups ranged from 123 to 246 per 100 000 and for the rest of the population 15 to 21 per 100 000. For schizophrenia, the rates for African–Caribbeans ranged from 33 to 108 and for the remaining population from 4 to 8 per 100 000.

Discussion

The researchers concluded that, despite the possibility of spurious results arising from the use of such low numbers of cases in their calculations, or from a possible underestimation of the African–Caribbean population, African–Caribbeans in Nottingham have a risk of psychosis and operationally defined schizophrenia up to eight times that of the remaining population. As this finding has been replicated consistently, they believe that the higher incidence found in African–Caribbeans has been established beyond reasonable doubt. The authors feel that it is now time to concentrate on investigating the aetiology of the disease, although they acknowledge that the small sample size in this and other research does not allow for adjustments to take account of socio-economic or other possible risk factors.

After a brief look at the evidence, hypotheses suggesting that the selective migration of vulnerable individuals and that genetic ethnic vulnerability is responsible for the phenomenon are discounted. The researchers conclude that a multi-factorial model best describes the aetiology of these psychoses and that the results can be explained by a coincidence of risk factors, such as prenatal or childhood infections, that come together because of the experience of migration.

Hatfield, B., Mohamad, H., Rahim, Z. & Tanweer, H. (1996) Mental health and the Asian communities: a local survey. *British Journal of Social Work*, **26**, 315–336.

Introduction

Concerns have been expressed about the experiences of Black and ethnic minority people with mental health problems. Studies investigating the incidence of mental health problems in the Asian community have produced mixed and sometimes contradictory results. Attention has been drawn to the need to address issues of cultural understanding and different (i.e. non-Western) perspectives on mental health. A review of hospital admission records of Asian people, living in the northern metropolitan borough of Milltown, had identified a small excess of psychiatric admissions and an excess of compulsory detentions. In addition, Asians appeared to be under-represented among those in receipt of community services. The study explores the views and experiences, in relation to mental health issues, of Asian people in the Milltown area.

Method

After a preliminary literature search, a questionnaire was devised to collect information about Asian people's constructions of mental health and mental illness, their views on appropriate responses/treatments, and their perceptions of appropriate services; in addition, their views on the availability and accessibility of services and cultural acceptability of services provided were sought. A mental health screening tool, the Langnez 22, was also completed by each subject. Subjects were randomly selected (using a population age quota system) from current and recent users of mental health community services and from Asian members of the public (recruited through mosques, community centres and so on).

Results

Among the 106 people interviewed, the most commonly cited stressors were: lack of official support, crime and personal safety, unemployment, financial problems and anxieties about children. Language difficulties, unemployment, physical illness, other family problems, lack of friends and relatives nearby and lack of official support were more prevalent among users of mental health services. Respondents as a whole seemed to experience relatively high levels of stress. Although 63% reported experiencing some form of hostility, disrespect or intolerance by the White community, this was not specifically related to mental health service use.

In response to questions about what caused mental health problems, the three most common answers were: social stress (87%), family problems (54%) and the will of God (34%). With regard to appropriate treatments, there was considerable support for counselling or support for people with mental health problems and support and advice for their families. Men were more likely to view Western medicine positively but also to favour complementary medicine. Treatment responses based on Islam were favoured by all Muslims. The need to address social problems was also raised.

Issues affecting the acceptability of services included the provision of appropriate diet, prayer facilities, washrooms, books and films, and single-gender facilities. Culturally-sensitive counselling was desired. There were preferences for staff of the same race and religion, and speaking the same language as service users, as well as for women staff for women users. Communication with White professionals was a widespread problem. A brief review of service users' contact with community professionals revealed that nearly 70% never saw a psychiatric nurse or other community health professional; in most cases follow-up support was provided by general practitioners.

Discussion

Higher levels of unemployment and housing disadvantage experienced by Asians in the Milltown area were not reflected by substantially higher hospital admission rates.

As expected, many of the sample viewed mental ill health in holistic terms, incorporating body and spiritual/religious dimensions, but not all. Religious explanations ranked highly as casual factors but other stressors were seen as more important. The interviews confirmed the need for more community-based support for mental health service users and their families – there was no evidence of the community having insular attitudes to care. The research highlighted the important role played by general practitioners in providing mental health services to this community.

Hemsi, L. K. (1967) Psychiatric morbidity of West Indian immigrants. *Social Psychiatry*, **2**, 96–100.

Introduction

The 1961 census confirmed West Indians as the largest single ethnic immigrant group in the UK. Despite this, relatively little demographic information was available about them. Studies of general practice attendance for mental disorders indicated that West Indian men were less likely and West Indian women twice as likely to present than their White counterparts, despite a higher prevalence of mild psychiatric problems in West Indians of both genders (although the higher rates were not found to be significant for men). The 1961 census made it possible for meaningful comparisons between ethnic groups to be made in respect of more serious mental health problems.

Method

The records of all first admissions to the seven psychiatric hospitals in the Camberwell and Lambeth catchment areas in London in 1961 were examined. However, only those patients without a previous psychiatric history who were between the ages of 15 and 54 years were included in the study. According to the 1961 census, over 90% of the West Indian immigrants living in the catchment areas were in this age range compared with some 53% of the indigenous population. Medical records were used to classify patients into two groups (native-born or West Indian) and to assign a diagnosis of schizophrenia, affective disorder, character/psychoneurotic disorder, organic syndrome or alcoholism/drug dependence.

Results

First-admission rates were considerably higher for West Indians (31.1 per 10 000) across all diagnoses compared with the native population (10.9 per 10 000). However, there were only 40 West Indian patients in the sample, and the total was broken down by gender and diagnosis. None of the West Indian patients were thought to have an organic mental illness or drug/alcohol dependence. Among the native population the incidence rates for both these diagnoses was very small, with the latter being non-existent in native women. Schizophrenia was the most common diagnosis for West Indian men, with an incidence rate of 13.1/10 000, compared with 2.7 for native men and 5.1 for West Indian women. The combined rate for affective disorders among West Indian men and women was 14.2 compared with 3.9 for the native population – these disorders were more often to be found in women than men.

Thus the West Indians differed from the native population in the rate and distribution of psychiatric disorders. A larger proportion were diagnosed with affective and schizophrenic disorders and a lower proportion with character, organic and drug- or alcohol-related disorders. Just over a quarter of the West Indian group were thought to have been ill on arrival in the UK or to have become ill soon afterwards. A further quarter became ill within two years, but the rest showed no sign of illness for two or more years after migration – 27% showed no significant illness for over four years after migration.

Discussion

The author begins by acknowledging the limitations of first-admission rates as measures of incidence, but feels that the differences found were so large that it is unlikely that the overall conclusions were not greatly affected. The results confirmed the finding of previous studies that migrant populations have higher rates of psychiatric morbidity than non-migrants. Only one study had investigated rates for West Indians in the West Indies and this had investigated rates only for psychosis. The differences between the incidence rates found were so large as to suggest that West Indian migrants have higher psychiatric morbidity than those who do not migrate. This finding was in line with a previous similar study looking at morbidity rates among Norwegian immigrants.

The researcher suggests that the time between migration and onset would suggest a causal relationship of some kind. In contrast to other research, the findings show higher incidence rates for West Indians with diagnoses of schizophrenia as well as affective disorder.

Hendricks, L. E., Bayton, J. A., Collins, J. L., Mathura, C. B., McMillan, S. R. & Montgomery, T. A. (1983) The NIMH Diagnostic Interview Schedule: a test of its validity in a population of black adults. *Journal of the National Medical Association*, **75**, 667–671.

Introduction

The National Institute of Mental Health (NIMH) in Washington, USA, developed the Diagnostic Interview Schedule (DIS) as a standardised tool for use in a series of multicentre epidemiological studies looking at the incidence and prevalence rates of specific mental disorders. The DIS, based on the DSM–III classification system, is intended to help researchers (from a variety of mental health disciplines) make consistent and accurate psychiatric diagnoses. The paper reports a pilot study examining its validity.

Method

After training, six medical students, two clinical psychology students and a medical social worker administered the DIS, along with the Centre for Epidemiological Studies Depression Scale (CES–D), to Black adults on low incomes who had been patients of Howard University Hospital and had a case note DSM–III diagnosis of depression, schizophrenia or alcohol dependency. Twelve patients with depression, 11 with schizophrenia and 23 alcoholic patients were included in the study.

Results

The DIS ratings of eight patients did not agree with the DSM–III diagnoses of schizophrenia made in their case notes. All eight were found to have a mixture of schizophrenic and depressive symptoms. Only in the case of one patient, who had recently stopped drinking, was the case note diagnosis of alcohol dependency not made on completion of the DIS. When it came to patients given a diagnosis of depression the DIS diagnosis exactly matched the case note information. These DIS ratings also compared well with CES–D scores. The researchers reported some difficulties in administering the DIS questionnaire, namely that it took too long to complete, it was difficult asking questions in the order specified and patients were uncomfortable answering some of the questions. The concordance for alcoholic patients and patients with depression was better than that for patients with schizophrenia.

Discussion

Only in the case of patients diagnosed with schizophrenia was agreement between case note and DIS information low. The authors suggest that this was owing to a lack of experience on the part of the raters. The difficulties experienced by raters in administering the DIS are thought to cast doubt on the content validity of the schedule for low-income Black respondents.

Hunt, N., Adams, S., Coxhead, N., Sayer, H., Murray, C. & Silverstone, T. (1993) The incidence of mania in two areas in the United Kingdom. *Social Psychiatry and Psychiatric Epidemiology,* **28,** 281–284.

Introduction

The incidence of mania ("the defining characteristic of bipolar disorder") in the inner-London borough of Hackney is compared with the incidence of mania in Chelmsford, a market town in southeast England. Hackney contains a relatively high number of recent immigrants from the New Commonwealth and is also considered one of the most socially disadvantaged boroughs in the UK. Chelmsford, on the other hand, is a relatively affluent rural area. The aim was to determine whether differences in socio-economic factors, ethnic origin or migration influence the rate of mania.

Method

The case notes of everyone aged 18–65 years living in the catchment area who had been admitted to psychiatric units within a two-year period were examined. Those with a likely diagnosis of bipolar affective disorder were invited for a clinical interview. If patients refused to be interviewed, information was obtained from relatives and medical personnel.

Results

The researchers found a substantial and significant difference between the two areas. While Chelmsford had a rate equivalent to the national average, Hackney's rate of mania was more than twice as high. The proportion of patients living in Hackney who were of UK/Irish origin, Caribbean origin or from the Indian subcontinent were approximately equal to that in the local population.

Discussion

The possibility that the different incidence rates for mania may have been due to differences in the threshold for admission in the two areas was considered and rejected. The age differences that existed between the two populations was also insufficient to account for the differences in incidence rates. Geographical mobility, however, was found to be significant. Few of the patients in Hackney were born in the area, whereas all but one of the Chelmsford patients was born locally. The researchers conclude that a mobile population has a higher risk of developing bipolar affective disorder. The relative affluence of the two areas is also thought to contribute significantly to the differences found.

Hutchinson, G., Takei, N., Bhugra, D., Fahy, T. A., Gilvarry, C., Mallett, R., Moran, P., Leff, J. & Murray, R. M. (1997) Increased rate of psychosis among African–Caribbeans in Britain is not due to an excess of pregnancy and birth complications. *British Journal of Psychiatry*, **171**, 145–147.

Introduction

It has been reported that pregnancy and birth complications (PBCs) increase the risk of schizophrenia for the infant. Some professionals have speculated whether an excess of PBCs can account for the greater incidence of schizophrenia found among African–Caribbeans in the UK. It is known that African–Caribbean and Asian women in England and Wales are more likely to die as a result of childbirth than women in the general population. In addition, African–Caribbean babies are two to three times more likely to be of low birth weight. It has been suggested that the enhanced survival of these babies contributes to the higher incidence of schizophrenia, particularly among second-generation African–Caribbeans. This study compares the prevalence rates of PBCs among African–Caribbean and White psychotic patients.

Method

Patients admitted to Bethlem and Maudsley hospitals between 1987 and 1993 were recruited to the study: if they were either White and British born or African–Caribbean and born in the UK or in the Caribbean; if they had a history of delusions, hallucinations, formal thought disorder or bizarre behaviour not due to organic factors; and if their mother was available to give obstetric histories.

Results

Of the 184 patients eligible, obstetric histories were available for 164 – 103 were White and 61 were African–Caribbean (30 of whom were first-generation migrants and 31 second-generation). Thirty-one patients (24 White and 7 African–Caribbean) had a history of PBCs. White patients were therefore almost twice as likely to have had PBCs, but this difference was not statistically significant. Neither was there any difference in the numbers of patients with a family history of psychosis, regardless of the presence or absence of PBCs. In relation to patients with schizophrenia only, 22 out of 114 had a history of PBCs (15 White and 7 African–Caribbean); the higher proportion of White patients was not statistically significant. As before, having a family history of psychosis was not found to be a significant factor either.

Discussion

The findings suggest that African–Caribbean patients were, if anything, less likely than their White counterparts to have had PBCs. This result was in line with other research which has indicated that African–Caribbeans are less likely to experience childhood neurological abnormalities and structural cerebral abnormalities – both possible consequences of PBCs.

Controversy exists over whether or not patients with schizophrenia without a family history of psychosis are more likely to have a history of PBCs. Although caution is needed because of the small sample size, the results here suggest that there might be some relationship, as none of the African–Caribbean patients who had experienced PBCs had relatives with a family history of psychosis.

Jablensky, A. (1995) Schizophrenia: recent epidemiologic issues. *Epidemiologic Reviews*, **17**, 10–20.

Introduction

This paper consists of a review of the literature about schizophrenia, in particular:

(a) new diagnostic systems and assessment instruments;
(b) new data on the frequency of schizophrenia, and its distribution within the population;
(c) new evidence and theories concerning risk factors;
(d) new studies of the course and outcome of schizophrenia.

Results

Populations with high incidence rates. Recent studies have uncovered very high rates of first admission with schizophrenia among African–Caribbean persons born in the UK. Errors in diagnosis and classification are now generally ruled out as explanations for this. A more recent study by King *et al* found higher incidence rates of schizophrenia among all ethnic minorities in the UK than among Whites. Comparable findings have been reported in the Netherlands. Explanations have tended to focus only on African–Caribbeans, and include possible overuse of cannabis, or a lower admission threshold for these people, but none of these propositions has been adequately tested. Another recent study has found a higher than expected risk of schizophrenia among the siblings of African–Caribbean probands with schizophrenia (born in the UK). This suggests that environmental factors are acting as triggers among those who have a genetic predisposition.

Decreasing incidence of schizophrenia. A number of studies published since 1985 have pointed to a fall in the first-admission rates for schizophrenia over the previous 30 years. However, the trend is not consistent within subgroups of the population, and has not been consistently replicated in local and regional data. Therefore, although the evidence is suggestive of a decline, the case is not yet proven. Jablensky adds that early reported rates may have been boosted by errors, and that only with the development of more sophisticated diagnostic instruments are true incidence rates being revealed.

Childhood precursors. A cohort study of children born in the UK found that children who went on to suffer from schizophrenia were more likely to experience speech and educational problems, and social anxiety, and were likely to prefer to play alone.

Cross-cultural comparisons. There is a large body of evidence from the World Health Organization that the course and outcome of schizophrenia are more likely to be positive in developing countries. The reasons for this are largely unknown. Jablensky suggests that they may be general, that is resulting from psychosocial factors such as beliefs and expectations, the presence of a social support network, or the existence of a non-stigmatising sick role in the early stages of illness. Alternatively, there may be as yet unidentified ecological factors at work (such as nutritional factors).

Discussion

The contribution of neurodevelopmental and environmental factors to the aetiology of schizophrenia is still unclear. Future research should give priority to discovering the effect of season of birth, the role of viral infection, the role of obstetric complications, the reason for the excess of schizophrenia among migrants and the reason for the suggested decline in incidence.

Jacob, K. S., Bhugra, D. and Mann, A. H. (1997) The validation of the 12-item General Health Questionnaire among ethnic Indian women living in the United Kingdom. *Psychological Medicine,* **27,** 1215–1217.

Introduction

The General Health Questionnaire (GHQ) has been validated in different cultures and in different languages including Kannada and Hindi in India. However, the validity of the 12-item GHQ (GHQ–12) has not been established among Indians resident in the UK.

Method

A consecutive sample of Indian women over the age of 16 presenting
to a general practice surgery were screened for psychiatric morbidity
using GHQ–12. A threshold of 1/2 was chosen and all those who
scored above the threshold and an equal number of individuals who
scored 0 or 1 were also interviewed using the Revised Clinical
Interview Schedule (CIS–R). Thresholds were compared against the
standard of the CIS–R.

Results

There were 48 GHQ-positive and 52 GHQ-negative subjects. The
optimal threshold for screening was found to be 2/3 with a positive
predictive value of 80.6% and a negative predictive value of 98.4%.
The sensitivity and specificity of the 2/3 threshold for Hindi speakers
was 94.1% and 91.7% respectively, and 100% and 88.2% for English
speakers.

Discussion

The results suggest that the threshold of 2/3 is more efficient for
screening whether Hindi or English versions are used for Indians in
the UK.

Jacob, K. S., Bhugra, D., Lloyd, K. & Mann A. H. (1998) Common
mental disorders, explanatory models and consultation behaviour
among Indian women living in the UK. *Journal of the Royal Society of
Medicine*, **91**, 66–71.

Introduction

Women of Indian origin are said to have lower rates of recognised
common mental disorders and a higher frequency of consultation
in primary care. This frequency of consultation may be related to
patients' beliefs regarding their illness. This study attempted to
examine the interrelationship between beliefs, common mental
disorders and consultation behaviour.

Method

In a large general practice in west London, a consecutive sample of
attenders who were female, originated from the Indian subcontinent,

and lived in the catchment area (but did not have psychosis, organic mental illness, learning disability or language disability) were approached to take part. The 12-item General Health Questionnaire (GHQ–12) was given to all subjects along with the Short Explanatory Model Interview (SEMI) and Revised Clinical Interview Schedule (CIS–R) to those who scored above 2 on GHQ–12.

Results

Of 140 patients contacted, 24 (17.1%) refused consent. A total of 100 patients were interviewed (48 GHQ-positive and 52 GHQ-negative). Thirty individuals (30%) met psychiatric case criteria (CIS–R threshold 12) and 29 (29%) met the ICD–10 diagnosis. Of these, 21 had depression, seven had neurasthenia and one had mixed anxiety and depression. Cases had a significantly higher consultation rate (9.3 per year compared with 4.6 per year for non-cases). The significant relation between frequency of consultations and psychiatric cases persisted even after adjustment for chronic physical illness, age, religion and marital educational and occupational status. Individuals who did not favour medical intervention had a significantly higher common mental disorders score even after adjustment on a number of variables and caseness. The general practitioner's (GP) recognition rate had a sensitivity of 17% and specificity of 91%. This was linked with whether patients told all their complaints to their GP. All non-cases said that they had discussed all their problems while only half of the 'cases' mentioned their problems to the GP. This difference remained significant even after age, education, occupation, marital status, religion, migrant status and total number of complaints were taken into account.

Psychiatric morbidity contributed to a high consultation rate in this population and yet a large number remained undiagnosed and untreated. The low level of patient perception of the need for medical treatment differs from the medical view that depression is an illness which requires intervention. Thus, most individuals who were cases did not disclose all their problems to their GP, leading to a possible under-recognition of psychiatric morbidity.

Discussion

The data on GP recognition were obtained from the case notes thus their reliability depends on whether the GP included all the information in the case notes. There was no control group to measure whether under-recognitioñ is the same in White patietnts.

King, M., Coker, E., Leavey, G., Hoare, A. & Johnson-Sabine, E. (1994) Incidence of psychotic illness in London: comparison of ethnic groups. *British Medical Journal,* **309,** 1115–1119.

Introduction

A large number of researchers have discovered higher rates of psychiatric admission to hospital, and higher rates of diagnosis for schizophrenia specifically, within the UK's African–Caribbean population than in the White community. This study aimed to determine the annual incidence and rate ratio of psychotic disorders in people from *all* ethnic groups resident in the catchment area under study.

Method

The researchers made contact with a wide range of community agencies, which were requested to provide details of all new cases of psychotic illness. The sampling frame included all individuals aged between 16 and 54 years who were resident in the catchment area and who came into contact with services between July 1991 and June 1992. Patients whose disturbances were clearly related to organic brain disease or to alcohol abuse were excluded. Patients who did fit the criteria were asked to take part in an interview in which the researchers gathered information about the patient's demographic characteristics, psychiatric history, current symptoms, help-seeking behaviour, drug use and ethnic group (using the categories of the 1991 census). A diagnosis was made using both ICD–9 and DSM–III criteria.

Results

Ninety-three persons were successfully recruited to the study (88% of those who met the entry criteria). There were no significant differences between the ethnic groups in terms of demographic characteristics, with the exception that the White patients were slightly older. The mean length of time between the onset of the disorder and the patient's first contact with services did not vary between ethnic groups. There was also no difference between the ethnic groups with respect to time taken for the illness to develop. There was a disproportionate number of Black patients among those with other less common psychotic disorders. All African–Caribbean patients with schizophrenia were under 29 years old, whereas there was a wider age range for other ethnic groups. No ethnic group was found to be significantly more likely to have been compulsorily admitted or to have been brought to the attention of services by the police.

Discussion

The annual incidence rate for schizophrenia found in this study was similar to that reported elsewhere. However, incidence rates of both schizophrenia and all other non-affective disorders were found to be higher among all the ethnic minorities than within the White sample. The researchers therefore suggest that it is wrong to view African–Caribbeans as particular victims of this illness, when in fact all ethnic minorities are at an increased risk. However, this research found that African–Caribbean patients developed schizophrenia at a younger age, although the lifetime prevalence of schizophrenia within this group may be closer to the rate within the wider population.

Koffman, J., Fulop, N. J., Pashley, D. & Coleman, K. (1997) Ethnicity and use of acute psychiatric beds: one-day survey in North and South Thames regions. *British Journal of Psychiatry*, **171**, 238–241.

Introduction

Migrants have often been found to experience higher rates of mental illness than members of the indigenous populations where they settle. Research in respect of African–Caribbeans in the UK has found over-representation in: psychiatric admissions; admissions under the Mental Health Act; admissions to secure units/special hospitals; and rates of schizophrenia. Explanations for these findings have been controversial. A one-day survey of acute adult and low-level secure psychiatric units in the North and South Thames regions provided the opportunity for the researchers to investigate the relationship between ethnicity and the use of psychiatric acute beds. The area surveyed contains 31 health authorities and has approximately 11 million adults.

Method

Ward managers in the regions' adult acute and low-level secure psychiatric units filled out forms on behalf of all in-patients, using their clinical notes. Information about patients' gender, age and ethnic group, mode of admission, type of ward and ICD–10 primary diagnosis was collected. Patients were divided into three ethnic groupings – White, Black and Asian – and census data adjusted for age and gender were used to calculate in-patient admissions ratios for each of these groupings.

Results

The survey identified 3710 adult acute and 268 low-level secure in-patients (out of a possible 3868 beds available). The sample was classified as 75% White, 16% Black and 4% Asian. (Of the private hospital patients surveyed, 23% were either Black or Asian.) Black patients were found to be over-represented in acute units. (Black psychiatric admissions ratios were calculated to be over four times that of the White population.) Moreover, 63.5% of Black patients were compulsorily detained compared with only 38.8% of the Asian patients and 30.6% of White patients. After controlling for diagnosis, the difference was still found to be significant. Of the Black patients, 10.5% were in low-level secure wards, compared with 3.1% of Asian patients and 6.1% of White patients – this difference was significant, as were differences in the proportions in each group who were not registered with a general practitioner. Black and Asian patients were significantly more likely to have a diagnosis of schizophrenia. However, no significant differences were found in the numbers of admissions patients had experienced in the previous 12 months.

Discussion

The authors acknowledge the methodological problems that might exist in this research, such as using 1991 census data to calculate ratios based on figures collected in 1994, when the profile of the local population may have changed in the intervening years. They also note that it would have been useful to have been able to control for socio-economic status. A number of factors have been thought to contribute to the over-representation of Black people within the mental health system. The authors suggest that the problem might in part reflect Black people's position in society (i.e. racism, poverty, etc.). Despite this, they feel that there are things that mental health practitioners can do to improve the situation, such as ask questions about access to services, about who receives what services and how, and about the appropriateness and quality of services (in particular, whether they meet the needs of local ethnic groups). They also say that the potential for discriminatory practices should be discussed openly.

Kulhara, P. (1994) Outcome of schizophrenia: some transcultural observations with particular reference to developing countries. *European Archives of Psychiatry and Clinical Neuroscience,* **224**, 227–235.

Introduction

Not until 1971 was the idea that the outcome of schizophrenia in non-White, non-European groups might be different from that in White Europeans explored in any depth. This paper reviews some of the work in this area.

Review

In 1971, Murphy & Raman reported that their follow-up of 90 Mauritian patients diagnosed with schizophrenia indicated that their outcome was better than that of UK patients followed up in a similar study carried out by Brown *et al* in 1966. These findings sparked much interest. However, Kulhara & Wig, in 1978, carried out a five-year study of patients in India and found that their sample had similar outcomes to patients in Brown *et al*'s study. Research carried out at about the same time in Sri Lanka tended to support the argument for a better outcome for non-Europeans. Kulhara & Wig suggested that the differing results were due to methodological inconsistencies.

Studies carried out by the World Health Organization (WHO) have used standardised assessment methods across the different countries. The WHO's International Pilot Study of Schizophrenia (IPSS) compared outcomes for schizophrenia across nine countries. Patients in the study were followed up one, two and five years after first contact. The results showed that at two- and five-year follow-up the outcome was more favourable for patients in developing rather than developed countries. Researchers in Colombia, one of the study centres, carried out a 10-year follow-up which showed the trend continuing.

The Determinants of Outcome of Severe Mental Disorders project (DOSMED), also carried out by the WHO, compared data across 12 centres in 10 countries. Patients with acute and insidious psychoses in developing countries did better than patients in more developed countries in the same category. Patients in developed countries spent proportionally more of the follow-up period experiencing psychotic episodes.

Subsequent independent research in India has not only confirmed the findings of the WHO studies but has additionally reported relatively low rates of social impairment among patients with schizophrenia. Studies carried out in Hong Kong and Singapore, although considered industrialised countries, are interesting because as Asian countries they may help to uncover the factors responsible for the differences in outcome. Unfortunately, these studies found contrasting results, most likely because of the use of different assessment techniques.

Discussion

Consideration is given as to whether the different outcomes could arise because comparisons were being made between different types of patients. For example, does the relative lack of mental health facilities in less developed countries mean that only people with the most florid symptoms come into contact with services? Differences in diagnostic procedures across countries that could have affected the results were also investigated, as some researchers had suggested that people in developing countries experiencing symptoms for a short time are given a diagnosis of schizophrenia when they would not in the West. However, earlier research by the author had found that, regardless of definition, patients in developing countries had a better outcome.

The author speculates that outcome is affected by as yet unspecified factors that vary from culture to culture. These factors may include: social acceptance of patients by the peer group; the social support networks available to the patient and family; family ties, structure and interactions; coping strategies of care givers; and 'expressed emotion' or guilt and hostility. Further exploration of the bio-sociocultural factors that influence outcome are needed to identify what actually is responsible for the better outcomes seen.

Leavey, G., King, M., Cole, E., Hoar, A. & Johnson-Sabine, E. (1997) First-onset psychotic illness: patients' and relatives' satisfaction with services. *British Journal of Psychiatry*, **170**, 53–57.

Introduction

It is thought that patients' and relatives' perceptions of services, at the time that psychotic disorders first becomes apparent, might affect compliance with care and clinical outcome. It has also been proposed by some researchers that dissatisfaction with services is one cause of the relatively poor compliance with care among Black patients. However, others have suggested that there is no great difference between Black and White patients' satisfaction with services. The aims of this study were: to assess satisfaction of patients and relatives with services after a first episode of psychosis; to examine factors associated with satisfaction; and to investigate any ethnic differences.

Method

Ninety-three patients within the catchment area of a north London hospital who were diagnosed, over a 12-month period, with a first-onset psychosis were approached to take part in the study. Patients completed questionnaires about their illness and, approximately a year after their first contact with services, they and their relatives were interviewed using specially designed service satisfaction questionnaires (one for patients and one for relatives). Questions were asked in relation to four domains of care:

(1) helpfulness of psychiatric care;
(2) information and advice;
(3) humane qualities of staff; and
(4) hotel aspects of hospital.

Relatives also completed the Family Service Satisfaction Scale (FSSS).

Results

Overall, services received relatively good approval ratings; however, patients and relatives were dissatisfied with the information given by staff about the illness and what to do in a crisis. Areas of low satisfaction in relation to the ward were to do with privacy, activities and contact with nursing staff. Relatives were less satisfied than patients in relation to time spent talking with doctors; doctors' explanations of treatment; sympathy and understanding of doctors; and information given on future crises. Patients born abroad were significantly more satisfied than those born in the UK on all four domains of care. Age, gender and diagnosis were not found to be related to satisfaction. Patients compulsorily detained were generally less satisfied than voluntary patients, but this was only significant in the case of domain 1. Relatives of sectioned patients were also significantly less satisfied in relation to domains 2 and 3. Relatives of patients diagnosed with schizophrenia were significantly less satisfied than others with domain 1. No significant differences were found in satisfaction levels between Black and non-Black patients on any of the four domains. Relatives of Black patients, on the other hand, were significantly more satisfied than others in relation to domain 4.

In relation to the FSSS, the relatives of Black patients were significantly more likely to answer 'none' when asked about assistance received in finding community care services or about participation in patients' treatment programmes.

Discussion

General statements appeared to elicit positive satisfaction ratings, but specific items produced more variable results. In line with other studies, communication between staff, patients and relatives was identified as a problem – no one staff member appeared to be responsible for sharing information. The FSSS also highlighted the way in which carers appeared to be excluded from decision making. The researchers found that the most significant variable in determining patient satisfaction was place of birth – the highest satisfaction was found among those born abroad. This could, the authors say, reflect lower expectations among this group. It is felt that the results of the study confirm similarities, in the initial stages of treatment, between different ethnic groups' experiences and perceptions of psychiatric services. This, along with Black patients' relatives' lower satisfaction with after-care, is in line with the view that the relationship between Black patients and psychiatric services tends to deteriorate over time, increasing the risk of involuntary admission.

Lindesay, J., Jagger, C., Mlynik-Szmid, A., Sonarwall, A., Peet, S. & Moledina, F. (1997) The Mini-Mental State Examination (MMSE) in an elderly immigrant Gujurati population in the United Kingdom. *International Journal of Geriatric Psychiatry*, **12**, 1155–1167.

Introduction

The Mini-Mental State Examination (MMSE) has been used extensively in epidemiological studies across different populations. The authors report on the validation of a version of MMSE as a measure of cognitive function and a screen for dementia in Gujurati elderly subjects.

Method

Designed as a two-stage community survey the authors identified elderly Asians and non-Asians from the register kept by the local Family Health Services Authority (FHSA), and subjects were contacted by post. The first-stage survey included information on demographic data, physical health problems, screening items for cognitive impairment and knowledge and use of community health and social services. Translated versions were employed. The second-stage survey involved interview by a psychiatrist to reach a clinical diagnosis as well as CAMCOG and SCAN instruments.

Results

A total of 207 Gujurati and 185 White subjects were sampled from the FHSA register and 28 and 20% respectively refused to participate. The Gujurati population was significantly younger than the White population. The Gujuratis had lower mean MMSE scores and these ethnic differences remained after adjustment for age group and educational differences (F=6.04, 1,287 d.f.; P<0.015). Visual impairment was more frequently reported by the Gujurati than the White subjects.

Overall, 74 Gujurati and 59 White subjects proceeded to the second stage of the study but only 27 and 42 respectively agreed to participate. Those who refused were most likely to be women and to have previously been a hospital out-patient. For all severities of dementia, rates in the Gujurati group were higher than in the White group.

Ethnic group only exerted a small independent effect on MMSE performance. The rates of dementia are higher among Gujuratis suggesting that this may be more common than previously reported. The large number of individuals refusing to take part, as well as other residential settings and longer delay in the Gujurati group between first and second stage, may well have influenced the rates.

Discussion

In spite of the small numbers, high non-responders and delay between two stages of surveys, this study suggests that rates of dementia in the Gujurati population are not as low as expected or previously reported. Even within the Gujurati version of the MMSE there remain serious problems about validating questions on orientation to time, place and person.

Lloyd, K. (1992) Ethnicity, primary care and non-psychotic disorders. *International Review of Psychiatry*, **4**, 257–266.

Introduction

This is a review of research into the primary care management of non-psychotic disorders such as anxiety and depression. There is a comparative lack of investigation in this area – most of the inter-ethnic research has concentrated on psychotic disorders and has been in relation to the African–Caribbean community.

Review

The author begins the review by investigating the relationship between ethnicity and registration with a general practitioner (GP). Previous reserach in the West Midlands, found that 99% of White, Asian and African–Caribbean households were registered with a GP. Most Asians had chosen to register with an Asian GP, most White patients with a White GP, with African–Caribbeans being more evenly spread. A look at research into GP attendance rates for various disorders found that men and women of Pakistani origin tended to have the highest number of consultations. Men of African–Caribbean and Indian origin also had significantly more consultations, while the women in these ethnic groups did not. A comprehensive study investigating GP consultations concluded that White patients consulted their GP most about psychological problems, while West Indians and Asian women consulted them the least. The author asks whether the different consultation rates found by researchers are due to differences in the prevalence of disorders. A review of the research in this area, however, produces conflicting results.

Studies that have tried to explain the relationship between ethnicity, gender, social class and support are also reviewed. Social differences, for example isolation and financial problems, are found to be associated with an increased prevalence of psychological problems. Women, it is said, are more likely than men to recognise minor emotional problems. However, Holland (1990) argued that the additive effects of gender, ethnicity and class reduce the likelihood of Black women seeking help for psychological problems.

The author attempts to investigate GPs' ability to detect psycho-logical problems in people of difference ethnic groups, but is hampered by a lack of research in this area. The question of somatic symptoms and their interpretation is also raised.

A brief look at studies into non-medical help-seeking is carried out in response to the suggestion that Black patients are more likely to seek help from sources other than medical professionals. But there is some evidence to suggest that White patients are just as likely to seek alternative sources of help. Some of the papers reviewed highlight distrust of health care and lifestyle and language barriers, lack of professional understanding and tolerance as reducing patients' willingness to seek help from a GP.

The possible role of discrimination and racism in relation to psychotic disorders is discussed. It has been argued that racism operates at many levels and in many ways in the delivery of services and that one way of combating it is to give ethnic minority consumers more control and choice in their treatment.

Discussion

The author concludes that relatively little is known about non-psychotic disorders and ethnic minorities. None of the explanations about why GPs are less likely to diagnose anxiety or depression in ethnic minorities than they are in the White population is found to be adequate. The need for more investigation is raised, as is the need to overcome reluctance by medical researchers to address issues of discrimination. Subjective experiences of services and the social context and history of ethnic minorities in the UK are felt to be important components of any future investigations.

Lloyd, K. (1993) Depression and anxiety among Afro-Caribbean general practice attenders in Britain. *International Journal of Social Psychiatry*, **39**, 1–9.

Introduction

Schizophrenia in African–Caribbeans in the UK, particularly the high prevalence rates found, has been the subject of much research. Biological and sociocultural reasons have both been put forward as possible explanations for higher rates, but it is the sociocultural explanations – such as social adversity, cultural mismatch of patients and doctors, culturally specific idioms of distress, unemployment and poor housing – that have found most favour. The same socio-cultural factors that are reported to affect rates of schizophrenia have also been associated with an increased risk of non-psychotic psychiatric disorders, such as depression and anxiety, most often seen by general practitioners (GPs). Yet the suggestion is that African–Caribbeans do not present to their doctors with these problems. Despite this anomaly, there has been relatively little research into the management of non-psychotic disorders in the UK African–Caribbean population. The author reviews the work that has been done in this area with the aim of explaining the apparent paradox.

Review

Evidence has shown that members of the UK's African–Caribbean population are just as likely to be registered with a GP as members of the White population. Although African–Caribbeans may tend to present to GPs with physical problems, research carried out in 1966, which suggested slightly higher attendance rates among this group, showed that GPs rated their conspicuous psychiatric morbidity as significantly greater than that of their White counterparts. More recent research has contradicted both aspects of this finding. A report of research carried out in 1989 indicated that, regardless of reason for consultation, White patients were more likely to leave the GP with a follow-up appointment, a prescription or a certificate. Studies comparing rates for minor psychiatric disorders among the African–Caribbean and White populations, although not clear cut, have tended to provide evidence for differences in consultation rates. It has been estimated that GPs detect only 60% of the psychiatric morbidity of their consulting population and that when the patient and doctor are from different cultural backgrounds this proportion is lower. Little has been done to discover whether there are differences between the ethnic groups in terms of the relationship between propensity to seek help and severity of symptoms. However, factors such as patients' attitudes to their health, distrust of the system, lifestyle and language barriers have all been shown to influence help-seeking. Many researchers have highlighted the fact that discrimination exists within health services, not just because of racist views of individuals but also as a consequence of institutional racism, which treats the beliefs, values and experiences of some people as inferior, bizarre or deviant.

Possible explanations are put forward for the relatively low rates of anxiety and depression found by GPs in African–Caribbean patients attending their surgeries. One possibility is that ethnic differences exist in the way in which the social precursors of schizophrenia may also operate for non-psychotic disorders. Another possibility is that African–Caribbeans do in fact experience lower rates of non-psychotic disorders than the general population. The author recommends that further epidemiological and anthropological studies are carried out in this area.

Lloyd, K. & Moodley, P. (1992) Psychotropic medication and ethnicity: an inpatient survey. *Social Psychiatry and Psychiatric Epidemiology*, **27**, 95–101.

Introduction

Numerous studies have shown that Black people's interaction with services can be different from that of their White counterparts, particularly in terms of the routes taken to in-patient care. Additionally, a higher proportion of Black people are diagnosed with schizophrenia. Questions have been asked about differences in treatment and in particular about whether differences exist in the management of Black people with schizophrenia, although previous studies in the UK have not always produced conclusive results. However, definite differences in after-care have been found. Against this background, this study investigated the use of medication in the treatment of Black and White in-patients in two south London hospitals.

Method

Demographic data, information about psychotropic medication prescribed, details of violent or self-harming behaviour and staff assessments of the risk of such behaviour were collected for all in-patients in the Bethlem and Maudsley hospitals. All data were amassed within five days of a designated census day, from a search of case notes, prescription cards and by interviewing primary nurses.

Results

Of the 145 possible patients in the sample, sufficient data were collected on 138 (37 of whom were Black and 101 of whom were categorised as non-Black). There were no differences found between the two groups in terms of age, gender, duration of admissions, length of time since first contact or number of admissions. The proportion of Black patients in the sample was not significantly different from their proportion in the general population of the catchment area. Although not over-represented among the in-patient population as a whole, 62% of Black patients had a diagnosis of schizophrenia compared with only 32% of the non-Black in-patients – making Black patients significantly more likely to have the diagnosis. They were also more likely to be on antipsychotic medication. Black patients were, however, significantly more likely to be on depot medication and, among these, Black patients were on significantly higher doses, although the wide range of doses used may have skewed results. Ethnicity ceased to be a significant variable in determining receipt of depot medication once diagnosis had been taken into account. None of the Black in-patients sampled were diagnosed with a neurotic illness.

Significantly more Black patients were found to have been detained under the Mental Health Act. Even after adjustments were made for variables such as diagnosis, ethnicity was still found to be a significant factor in determining the likelihood of compulsory detention.

Black patients were not rated by staff to be any more violent than their non-Black counterparts, despite being more likely to have been involved in violent incidents in both past and present admissions. There remained a significant relationship between a record of violence and ethnicity even when adjustments were made for confounding variables. Black patients were also more likely to have been on a locked ward in the past, although this did not hold true for the current admission.

Discussion

The large number of Black in-patients in the sample with a diagnosis of schizophrenia led the authors to question whether the findings were a result of general practitioners' failure to recognise non-psychotic disorders in Black people, or a result of Black people's failure to approach their general practitioners with these problems. The greater likelihood of Black patients receiving depot medication, and the higher doses they received, was thought to arise from a greater perceived risk of their non-compliance with oral medication. The author recommends that the relationship between ethnicity and compulsory detention is investigated further, as should be the relationship between ethnicity and in-patient violence. This is of particular interest because the same staff who were responsible for recording more violent incidents by Black in-patients actually perceived Black patients to be less likely to be involved in violence. Further work to investigate the relationship between Black patients' views of services and the attitudes and practices of non-Black care professionals is also recommended.

Lloyd, K. & Bhugra, D. (1993) Cross cultural aspects of psychotherapy. *International Review of Psychiatry*, **5**, 291–304.

Whether forms of psychotherapy which originated in the West can be employed without appropriate modification to other cultures remains a potent topic for debate. The universalist view that all individuals have more similarities than differences contrasts with the relativist view, which suggests that each culture is unique and cannot (and should not) be embraced by any general theory. The authors take a historical and political context within which psycho-therapy in particular and psychiatriatry in general have developed. The roles of ethnic matching and cultural matching of therapists and patients are discussed within the American context along with the application of such findings to British clinical practice. Ethnic matching can be a false solution and the whole being of the individual must be taken into account. The authors describe different forms of psychotherapy which have advantages and disadvantages for different minority ethnic groups. These therapies and indigenous therapies are illustrated with specific examples from the Indian subcontinent. The authors conclude that almost all therapy can and should be seen as a form of cross-cultural psychotherapy, and further-more, that clinicians should be self-reflexive and aware of their own prejudices, ideology and power.

Lloyd, K., Jacob, K. S., Patel, V., St Louis, L., Bhugra, D. & Mann, A. H. (1998) The development of the Short Exploratory Model Interview (SEMI) and its use among primary care attenders with common mental disorders. *Psychological Medicine,* **28**, 1231–1237.

Introduction

Explanatory models (EMs), defined as notions about an episode of sickness and its treatment, are important contributions to research into ethnic perspectives of illness. These include beliefs concerning the aetiology of the illness, its course, the timing of the symptoms, the meanings of sickness, its diagnosis and the methods of treatment, and the roles and expectations of the subjects involved in the process. The elicitation of the patient's EMs and the healer's understanding can help the patient make sense of his or her experience. Patterns of service utilisation may be important consequences of EMs.

Method

The Short Explanatory Model Interview (SEMI) has five sections which cover (a) personal, cultural and social background; (b) nature of problem, reasons for consultation, perceived causes, its effect on body, emotions, mobility, social network, home life, finances and work; (c) help-seeking – biomedical and alternative; (d) interaction with healers – role, expectation and satisfaction; and (e) beliefs related to mental health and illness.

Primary care attenders in west London, south London and Harare were approached to participate in the study. The interview was translated and back-translated into Shona and Hindi.

Results

Non-specific symptoms were more common in Harare and west London Asian samples. The Asians were more likely not to know the reasons for the onset of their symptoms compared to others, whereas Harare subjects attributed these to interpersonal and social as well as supranatural causes. Perceived seriousness of their problem was not significantly different in any of the groups. Expectation of learning the diagnosis and of receiving explanation and advice was most commonly seen among Whites, whereas Asians were much more likely to expect tablets and injections. A higher proportion of Zimbabweans and British African–Caribbeans reported believing in black magic and spells (65% and 39% respectively), compared with no Whites and only 11% Asians.

Two case vignettes of depression as psychological and somatisation were administered to the UK samples only. Asians were the least likely to see depression as psychological and to seek medical help for depression as well as somatisation.

The instrument is therefore valid in its capacity to identify variations in beliefs and expectations about illness and its treatment in a brief, efficient and reliable manner. The simplicity and brevity of the instrument allows for its use in field studies in different cultures and clinical settings.

Discussion

Due to the brevity of the instrument it cannot replace detailed anthropological enquiry and needs to be used in conjunction with clinical enquiry.

Lockhart, S. P. & Baron, J. H. (1987) Changing ethnic and social characteristics of patients admitted for self poisoning in West London during 1971/2 and 1983/4. *Journal of the Royal Society of Medicine,* **80,** 145–148.

Introduction

Ethnic minorities in inner-city areas face social, economic and cultural stresses which affect their mental health. A key idiom of distress under these circumstances can be attempted suicide. With time, social stresses changes and a change in rates of attempted suicide will be expected.

Method

Consecutive adults aged 15 or over admitted to a general hospital in west London were studied during two periods – first, November 1971 to February 1972, and secondly September 1983 to June 1984. For each patient, the physician completed a questionnaire. Data for the base population were obtained from the census.

Results

During the first period, 93 patients were admitted on 100 occasions from a catchment population of 92 720. During the second, 86 patients were admitted on 94 occasions from a catchment population of 73 929. The population of West Indians rose from 0 to 7% – a significant increase – whereas there was a significant fall in the White population. The social classes 4 and 5 increased from 39% to 48% between the two periods. Level of use of barbiturates as a drug for overdose fell but that of paracetamol increased over the same period.

Discussion

The most striking finding was the fall in the number of admissions between 1971 and 1984 which may reflect changes in admission policy, change in base population and other factors. The other significant finding was the increase in the number of West Indians attempting suicide, which the authors attribute to possible assimilation of European values and attitudes because there were more socio-demographic similarities with the White group. The significant fall in the number of patients claiming prior psychiatric care suggests that other factors may be at play in precipitating attempted suicide.

Although the numbers are small, changes in findings according to the period of comparison do suggest that several complex factors are at play in contributing to attempted suicide.

McGovern, D. & Cope, R. (1991) Second generation Afro-Caribbeans and young whites with a first admission diagnosis of schizophrenia. *Social Psychiatry and Psychiatric Epidemiology*, **26**, 95–99.

Introduction

Previous studies investigating the prevalence of schizophrenia among African–Caribbeans had tended to concentrate on the rates for first-generation immigrants. In this study, the researchers investigate the first-admission rates of second-generation African–Caribbeans admitted to a Birmingham hospital from 1980 to 1982.

Method

African–Caribbean patients aged 16–29 years were categorised as second-generation migrants for the purposes of the study. The case notes of these African–Caribbean patients who had a first-admission diagnosis of schizophrenia, along with those of White patients of similar age and circumstance, were examined. As a result, 29 White patients and 33 African–Caribbean patients were included in the study. Demographic data and details of diagnoses, such as the presence of first-rank symptoms and individual psychosocial stressors relevant to the onset of symptoms, were collated, along with information about the mode of admission, any services patients had had contact with, mode of discharge and follow-up arrangements.

Results

Significant differences between African–Caribbean and White patients were few. However, significantly more African–Caribbeans lived alone. Differences in the rate of onset of symptoms (which was faster for African–Caribbeans) almost reached significance, as did differences in contact with services before admission – African–Caribbeans were less likely to have seen their general practitioner and more likely to have had contact with the police or prison services. African–Caribbeans' follow-up attendance was likely to be more sporadic, but this difference also was not quite significant.

Discussion

The researchers acknowledge that the small sample size made it difficult for them to achieve statistically significant results. They speculate about why more African–Caribbeans in the study were single. Is this something that is true for the African–Caribbean population as a whole, or only for those diagnosed with a mental illness? The problems of labelling theory as an explanation for excessive diagnosis of schizophrenia in African–Caribbeans is discussed. If, as labelling theory suggests, being Black and single provides an increased risk of being labelled then it follows that there should be large numbers of White people undiagnosed. The authors disagree with this hypothesis. They also found little evidence of inappropriate diagnosis. They suggest one explanation for their findings is that economic hardship made it more difficult for people who are ill to live with their families. They propose that it is the fact of being unemployed, single and living alone that leads to patients follow a different pathway to services.

The authors note the link found between African–Caribbeans and the forensic system, but feel this is better discussed elsewhere. On every measure African–Caribbeans were less likely to make voluntary contact with services. They conclude that African–Caribbeans find psychiatric services less satisfactory and relevant to their needs than their White counterparts.

McGovern, D. & Hemmings, P. (1994) A follow-up of second generation African–Caribbeans and white Britons with a first-admission diagnosis of schizophrenia. Attitudes to mental illness and psychiatric services of patients and relatives. *Social Science and Medicine*, **38**, 117–127.

Introduction

Many previous research studies had found that African–Caribbeans experience higher rates of schizophrenia. This has been true of studies investigating rates in both first- and second-generation migrants. Indeed, some evidence suggests even higher rates among second-generation African–Caribbeans. Differences with Whites have also been found in the routes African–Caribbeans take to services – they are less likely to have had contact with their general practitioner, more likely to have had contact with the police or prison services and less likely to have had voluntary contact with services. Some researchers have also suggested that the quality of care offered to Black patients is inferior – for example, that they are more likely to be given physical treatments or to be seen by junior doctors. Some recent studies, however, found contrary evidence.

In this light, the authors investigated African–Caribbeans' attitudes to care and satisfaction with services.

Method

African–Caribbean and White patients aged 16–29 years admitted to a Birmingham psychiatric hospital between 1980 and 1984 with a first-admission diagnosis of schizophrenia were interviewed in 1989 as part of a follow-up study (see McGovern *et al*, 1994, below). A close relative or partner was also interviewed, where possible. A combination of standard questionnaires such as the Client Satisfaction Questionnaire (CSQ8) and specifically designed Likert scales were used.

Results

Of the 33 original White patients in the sample, 28 were included in the follow-up study, and of the 42 original Black patients, 37 were included. No significant differences were found between the two groups in terms of: global satisfaction and satisfaction with individual domains of health care – although the less satisfaction felt by Black patients over whether or not they saw their preferred staff member was almost significant; the way in which patients conceptualised their problems as a mental illness; whether or not relatives felt patients were responsible for their symptoms; and patients' views of psychiatric treatment.

Statistical differences were found in some areas, however. More Black relatives felt that substance misuse was a causal factor in the development of their relatives' problems. Black patients and relatives were also significantly more likely to believe that Black people were not treated as well as Whites by services or else were not sure about this. The preference of Black patients to be followed up on discharge at home and the preference for White patients to be followed up in non-psychiatric health settings was not quite significant. Neither were differences in beliefs about the usefulness of specialist day centres – Black patients and relatives tended to believe that Black day centres benefit Black patients.

Discussion

The sample is small and the attitudes were measured several years into contact with services. As the authors acknowledge, either the chronic course of problems itself or repeated contact with psychiatric services may well have influenced their views. The attitudes to cannabis are interesting. The differences in treatment compliance are unlikely to be explained by differences in attitudes to treatment. The authors conclude that contrary to expectation, their study showed little difference between the two groups.

McGovern, D., Hemmings, P., Cope, R. & Lowerson, A. (1994) Long-term follow-up of young Afro-Caribbean Britons and white Britons with a first admission diagnosis of schizophrenia. *Social Psychiatry and Psychiatric Epidemiology*, **29**, 8–19.

Introduction

Some researchers have suggested that in recent years there has been an increase in the incidence of schizophrenia among young African–

Caribbeans in the UK. This study investigated whether "a diagnosis of schizophrenia has the same implications for Black and White people in terms of outcome and response to treatment".

Method

The sample consisted of Black and White patients with a diagnosis of schizophrenia. All lived in the catchment area of a Birmingham hospital, were first admissions and were aged 16–29 years. Patients, their relatives and the professionals involved were all interviewed and case notes examined. The minimum follow-up period after admission for patients in the sample was just under 5 years and the maximum 10 years.

Results

Thirty-three White patients and 42 Black patients were followed up. The researchers found no difference between the two groups in terms of the validity of the diagnosis of schizophrenia. However, Black patients had significantly more readmissions in the follow-up period. Black patients were also more likely to have had convictions and to have been imprisoned. There were significantly more Black admissions under part III (forensic sections) of the Mental Health Act and in readmissions from prison. None of the other differences in treatment or outcome measures was significant.

Discussion

The researchers indicate that possible reasons for the poor prognosis of Black patients may include the negative effects of labelling. In other words, it seems that a diagnosis of schizophrenia has more negative effects on Black than on White patitnts. Characteristics of the patient group were also thought to have affected outcome, but only socio-economic differences were found. There did not appear to be any differences in the illness itself that would account for differing prognoses. The only difference found in relation to treatment adequacy was the higher compulsory admission rates among the African–Caribbean sample. However, the researchers were not able to consider qualitative differences such as patient satisfaction, concepts of illness and attitudes to care.

Investigation of the psychosocial factors affecting patients showed that Black patients were more likely to be living alone – possibly due to the effects of migration or socio-economic hardship. They were also more likely to have been imprisoned and to have a poor record of employment. All these factors have, in the past, been associated with poor prognosis. The researchers conclude that these social factors best explain the differences found and that a reduction in these handicaps would reduce differences in outcome.

McKeigue, P. M. & Karmi, G. (1993) Alcohol consumption and alcohol-related problems in Afro-Caribbeans and South Asians in the United Kingdom. *Alcohol and Alcoholism,* **28,** 1–10.

Introduction

This review analyses the literature about alcohol consumption by African–Caribbeans and South Asians in the UK. The term African–Caribbean is used to refer to people of African descent from the American New Commonwealth and the term South Asian to refer to people from India, Pakistan, Bangladesh, Sri Lanka and Nepal. All of the three main religions in this region prohibit the use of alcohol but only among Muslims is the principle widely adhered to.

Alcohol and African–Caribbeans

Surveys in the UK in the 1970s and '80s have consistently shown lower average alcohol consumption and heavy drinking by African–Caribbeans compared with their White counterparts. National data show that death rates from chronic liver disease and cirrhosis are no higher among African–Caribbeans than the national average, whereas among the Irish- and South-Asian-born men rates are higher. Studies suggest that for African–Caribbeans alcohol misuse is a less common cause of admission to general hospitals than it is for the White population.

Alcohol and South Asians

The authors examine the alcohol consumption of the three main religious groups in South Asia: Hindus, Sikhs and Muslims. The studies involving Gujarati Hindus all show considerably lower rates of alcohol consumption for this group than for the White population. Investigations into alcohol consumption among Sikhs do not show their consumption to be significantly greater than that of the White population, although the profile of drinking is slightly different – Sikh heavy drinkers tend to be older men and to drink alone. The lowest rates of alcohol consumption can be found among Muslims, and Bangladeshi Muslims appear to drink the least.

Analysis of studies into alcohol-related deaths and liver disease among people of South Asian origin indicates higher rates than would be expected. This suggests that South Asians are more vulnerable than Europeans to alcohol-induced liver damage, but no studies have been carried out to confirm this.

A national survey carried out in 1971 identified that psychiatric admissions for alcohol-related problems were higher in Indian-born men and all South Asian-born women than for the UK-born population. Other studies have suggested that serious alcohol problems are especially common among Sikh men.

Service provision and prevention

Alcohol advisory services report seeing few Black clients even when located in areas with a high ethnic minority population – although a few specialist services aimed specifically at South Asians do exist. The authors report that the Health Education Authority Alcohol Programme has few materials aimed at ethnic minority groups.

Discussion

The authors point out that despite lower rates of heavy drinking among African–Caribbeans, alcohol-related psychiatric admissions are rising and the numbers of deaths from hypertension and stroke are relatively high. So, a rise in consumption levels to those of the native population could have serious consequences.

The average alcohol consumption rates for Gujarati Hindus, Muslims and all South Asian women is relatively low, although heavy drinkers exist in all groups, especially among Sikh men. South Asians have relatively high rates of alcohol-related psychiatric admissions and high death rates from chronic liver disease.

The authors suggest that future research should monitor secular trends in alcohol consumption because alcohol-related problems seem to be increasing relatively quickly in some minority groups. Beliefs, attitudes and behaviour in respect of alcohol use (in the Sikh community in particular) need to be investigated.

Mathers, D. C. & Ghodse, A. H. (1992) Cannabis and psychotic illness. *British Journal of Psychiatry*, **161**, 648–653.

Introduction

The researchers point out that the dramatic changes in behaviour and perception produced by cannabis have been reported since 3000

BC. The increased use of cannabis in America after prohibition led to the La Guardia Commission (1944) in which they did not find a link between cannabis use, crime and insanity. Despite this, anecdotal reports have linked acute intoxication with confusional states and transient psychosis, and intoxication has been said to exacerbate underlying neurotic problems. Mania, depression, schizophrenia and mixed psychotic states have all been linked to 'cannabis psychosis'. Some researchers have suggested that cannabis users come from a group in the population that is already at high risk of developing a psychiatric illness. Other research has been criticised for assuming that correlation implies cause. The authors investigated the relationship further by looking at the natural history of cannabis use and psychosis.

Method

Patients admitted to an acute ward of a south London hospital between August 1986 and February 1988 were interviewed to determine the presence of psychotic symptoms and use of cannabis, alcohol or illicit drugs before admission. Urine samples were also collected. The sample comprised patients aged 16–60 years who had psychotic symptoms and did not misuse alcohol or use illicit drugs other than cannabis. All cannabis users were included, and every eighth patient who met the criteria but who did not use cannabis was selected for the control group. Sixty-one subjects and 43 controls were interviewed, using the Present State Examination (PSE), a week after admission and again one month and six months later. Urine samples were also repeated. In addition, demographic information and drug use history were collected.

Results

Subjects tended to be younger than controls, and more of them were male; more cannabis users were non-White and had a history of psychotic illness, a forensic history and a past compulsory admission. A PSE comparison of the two groups showed differences in changed perception, non-verbal auditory hallucinations, thought insertion, delusions of control and delusion of grandiose ability at one week. At one month, differences were found in only one item – delayed sleep. At three months no differences were found.

The PSE variables also differed for Black and White patients at one week. White patients tended to experience sleep delay, early-morning waking, loss of libido, flight of ideas and obsessional checking. Black patients tended to have culturally influenced delusions. When Black patients were removed from the comparison between subjects and controls, only two areas of difference previously identified remained significant – level of non-verbal auditory hallucinations and delusions of control. Three new items became significant – feelings of hopelessness, derealisation and depersonalisation.

Discussion

Of 140 PSE items, in only five were significant differences found between the two groups at one week. These differences could therefore have been due to chance, but because earlier studies had found differences in similar areas the authors do not feel this to be the case. They point to the need to determine whether symptoms are dose-related. However, subjects were unwilling to provide this information, so it was not possible to explore this.

Factors that could explain why Black cannabis users were more psychotic and less anxious or depressed include: amount taken, setting in which the drug was used or the lack of cultural mediation in the case of the White sample. More investigation is needed, especially as the sample and controls were not a homogeneous group. The authors also point out that cannabis use may be a marker for marginalisation. Their findings suggest that an acute psychotic episode following cannabis use may be more likely if there is a history of psychotic disorder.

The authors recommend routine urine screening in patients aged under 35 with psychosis – feeling that this would help to clarify the effect of this relatively commonly used drug.

Moodley, P. & Perkins, R. E. (1991) Routes to psychiatric inpatient care in an inner London borough. *Social Psychiatry and Psychiatric Epidemiology*, **26**, 47–51.

Introduction

Research into pathways to care has tended to concentrate on referrals to services generally. This study investigates referral routes to inpatient services specifically. The research was carried out in a deprived inner-London borough, with a relatively high proportion (23%) of the population being from ethnic minorities – mainly of African–Caribbean origin.

Method

Basic demographic information, referral routes, psychiatric history and diagnoses were collected from 60 consecutive adult admissions to psychiatric wards serving the relevant catchment area. Fifty-two of the patients agreed to be interviewed. Interviews were carried out within a week of admission.

Results

The majority of the sample interviewed were young, single, unemployed, living in council accommodation and had had previous admissions. The sample was 48% White and 42% of African–Caribbean origin. African–Caribbean patients tended to be younger, but their demographic details were otherwise similar to those of the White patients. African–Caribbeans aged over 30 years were more likely to receive a diagnosis of psychosis. A high proportion of older Whites had a diagnosis of depression. A similar proportion of Black and White patients reported social and psychiatric difficulties, but a higher proportion of White people reported physical problems or had taken overdoses. A higher proportion of African–Caribbeans thought they did not have a problem.

The sample had taken a variety of routes to in-patient care. The largest proportion (38.4%) had came straight to psychiatric care either on their own volition or at the insistence of friends or relatives. This represented 40% of people under 30 but only 10% of people over 30. Overall, 23.1% of the sample came via the police or legal system: this represented 40% of people under 30 and 16.7% of people over 30. People over 30 were most likely to come to in-patient services via general hospital services or through psychiatric out-patient departments. There were no significant gender differences or differences between African–Caribbeans and Whites in terms of the routes they took.

Overall, 40.4% of the sample had been compulsorily detained, but a significantly higher proportion of African–Caribbeans (59%) were so compared with White patients (24%). Fifty per cent of patients diagnosed with manic depression, 57% of those with schizophrenia or schizoaffective disorder and 7.7% of those suffering depression were compulsorily detained. Linear logistic analysis showed that although African–Caribbeans were more likely to be diagnosed with psychotic disorders, it was their ethnic status rather than their diagnosis that made them more likely to be compulsorily detained.

Discussion

A relatively small proportion of patients came to in-patient services through their general practitioner (GP). According to the researchers, this could be either because most of the patients who keep in contact with their GP have the support they need to keep out of hospital or because the sample did not feel that GPs were an appropriate source of help. They postulate that for 'revolving door' patients, specialist outreach and continuing care services are a more appropriate form of community support than the GP.

The high level of police involvement in referrals led the researchers to conclude not only that services were failing younger patients but also that police involvement led to an unwillingness on behalf of patients to engage with services in the future. They recommend the development of 24-hour emergency walk-in services, as this was a resource that was well used by the younger age group, despite being located outside the catchment area. Additionally, very few of the patients admitted were in contact with community mental health workers and several had reported problems getting appropriate help. The researchers conclude by saying that accessibility and availability of services may be the key to improving community-based support.

Morley, R., Wykes, T. & MacCarthy, B. (1991) Attitudes of relatives of Afro-Caribbean patients: do they affect admission? *Social Psychiatry and Psychiatric Epidemiology*, **26**, 187–193.

Introduction

High rates of compulsory admission have been reported among African–Caribbean patients when compared with White patients. It has been suggested that the difference in rates might be accounted for by the excess of admissions for schizophrenia. Other possible explanations involve allegations of racism in the provision of psychiatric services. Violence has also been cited as a reason for the levels of compulsory detention. Some have suggested that African–Caribbean relatives are more likely to perceive the disturbed family member as being dangerous – thus lending credence to the perceptions of admissions staff. This study set out to explore whether the high rates of African–Caribbean patients compulsorily admitted to hospital can be explained by the attitudes of relatives.

Method

African–Caribbean patients admitted consecutively to psychiatric units covering three inner-London health districts and who were reportedly experiencing psychotic symptoms were identified, and those in close contact with a relative or partner were interviewed using the Present State Examination. The close relative or partner was interviewed using a range of questionnaires.

Results

Ten informally admitted patients and 15 compulsorily detained patients and their key relatives participated in the study. Seventy-six per cent of the sample had had one previous admission. Seventy-six per cent had been born in the West Indies, but had lived in the UK for over 20 years. Thirty-six per cent were diagnosed with schizophrenia and the remaining with one of the following: paranoid psychosis, manic psychosis or borderline psychosis. There was no evidence that those who had been compulsorily detained were more ill than the others.

Twice as many relatives of detained patients thought that their relative was not a danger to themselves or to others. There was no support for the hypothesis that a legal model was held more often by relatives of detained patients. There was also no support for the prediction that relatives of detained patients had a more negative opinion of psychiatric services.

Discussion

The authors acknowledge that their sample was small and that there was a high drop-out rate, but they do not believe that any significant biases were introduced as a result. None of the expected differences between the two groups of patients in terms of severity of illness and dangerousness was found. Furthermore, none of their hypotheses concerning the attitudes of relatives contributing to the likelihood of compulsory admission was supported either. More investigation is recommended into whether or not staff expectations of increased violence from African–Caribbean patients are unfounded. The question of whether psychiatric services are more reluctant to become involved with African–Caribbean families or to provide African–Caribbean patients with informal treatment is also raised by the authors.

Moselhy, H. F., McKnight, A. & Macmillan, J. F. (1995) The challenge of self-mutilation. A case report and review of literature. *European Journal of Psychiatry*, **9**, 161–165.

Introduction

Self-mutilation is common among young adult patients with personality disorder. It can also be seen in patients with psychosis, who tend to exhibit more severe forms of self-mutilation, possibly while acting under some delusional belief involving body parts. The author describes the case of a 22-year-old African–Caribbean man with schizophrenia who tried to amputate his right hand with a saw (removing three fingers and half of his palm in the attempt). He told staff when subsequently admitted to psychiatric hospital that his right hand should be cut off as a punishment for having 'sinned against God, at the age of 15, by attempting suicide.

Case report

The patient was admitted to psychiatric hospital for the first time at 20, also for attempting to cut off his right hand. He was the fourth of six children; his parents (both still alive) were separated. His mother and elder brother had both been diagnosed with schizophrenia; his brother committed suicide at 27. His sister also had contact with services. The suicide attempt, an overdose, came about after an argument with his mother, who he felt preferred his younger brother and did not love him. Following this attempt he became isolated. He had never had any significant sexual relationships.

On admission the patient denied hallucinations, but exhibited bizarre behaviour, such as emptying salt cellars into his food and unprovoked aggressive outbursts. After being prescribed zuclopenthixol his behaviour became more sociable and less bizarre and he was discharged after nine months. He was admitted again two weeks later, after successfully amputating most of his right hand. He was unwilling to talk about his beliefs and about why he had amputated his hand. In spite of large doses of neuroleptics this refusal continued, as did his bizarre behaviour. Consequently, he was prescribed clozapine. Because of a change in hospital catchment areas, after five months he was transferred to another hospital, where he confided in African–Caribbean staff members that he had deliberately hurt himself and wondered if he had misread the biblical text, but he did not regret his act. He also talked about abusive auditory hallucinations and delusions of control.

He was subsequently discharged to an African–Caribbean residential home, where he continued to see a psychologist. His social interaction at the time was appropriate, although he still remained deluded and was regarded as being at high risk of further self-mutilation.

Discussion

Similar studies have described self-mutilation in psychotic patients in psychoanalytic terms (e.g. as being due to unresolved Oedipal conflicts, repressed homosexual impulses, severe guilt, self-punishment or religious delusions). Researchers have also pointed to a previous act of self-mutilation and delusions as significant factors in predicting further self-mutilation.

Some researchers had concluded that cultural beliefs must in some way serve to protect or aggravate severe self-destructive behaviour, because it is so rarely reported in developing countries. Other researchers have suggested that severe self-mutilation does occur as commonly in developing countries and that there are no cultural beliefs affecting such behaviour. This is in contrast to this study, where religious beliefs and cultural distance prevented communication between staff and patient. The author emphasises that it was some five months later, to a psychologist and nurse of the same cultural background, that the patient confessed his delusions. The conclusion is that cultural distance was probably an important factor preventing the prediction of severe self-mutilation.

Nayani, S. (1989) The evaluation of psychiatric illness in Asian patients by the Hospital Anxiety and Depression Scale. *British Journal of Psychiatry*, **155**, 545–547.

Introduction

Evidence from transcultural psychiatry has implied similar rates of psychiatric morbidity in both Western and non-Western countries. However, some conditions are said to have different cultural clinical presentations. While some have said that Asians somatise depressive symptoms, others have disagreed. This study examined the usefulness of the self-assessment Hospital Anxiety and Depression scale (HAD) for Asian patients and at the same time investigated psychological and somatic expressions of patients' symptoms.

Method

Urdu-speaking Asian patients, aged 16 and over, attending the Transcultural Psychiatric Clinic in Bradford were asked to complete an Urdu version of the HAD. Patients with organic or psychotic illness were excluded. The Clinical Interview Schedule (CIS) was administered by a bilingual psychiatrist. The CIS consists of 10 reported symptoms (depression, anxiety, somatic symptoms, etc.) and 12 manifest abnormalities, each rated on a five-point scale. HAD detects a possible case (cut-off 7 or 8) or probable case (cut-off 10 or 11) for each of the two scales. The present study compared the cut-off score of 7 or 8 with a CIS score of 2 or above on each symptom rating for case identification.

Results

Nine men and 11 women aged 25–58 years took part in the study. All were semi-skilled workers with some formal education who had had their symptoms for a mean of 4.7 years.

The somatic and anxiety scores on both the HAD and CIS were found to be significantly correlated. However, depression ratings were not. The HAD depression subscale had greater specificity (70%) and sensitivity (85%) than the anxiety subscale (with a specificity of 37.5% and a sensitivity of 66%).

Discussion

Somatic symptoms were found to be related to anxiety but not depression. Correlations between the HAD and CIS scores were low. The authors hypothesise that the CIS distinguished between somatic and anxiety symptoms but the HAD did not. So the HAD could not identify patients with anxiety according to CIS criteria, but it could identify patients with depression.

The author concluded that it is possible to detect depressive illness in Asian patients using the translated HAD, but that it should not be used as a screening instrument for anxiety. The author notes that the translators of the HAD into Urdu were careful to focus on concepts rather than producing an exact literal translation of each sentence.

Noble, P. & Rodger, S. (1989) Violence by psychiatric in-patients. *British Journal of Psychiatry*, **155**, 384–390.

Introduction

In 1976 the Bethlem and Maudsley hospitals started a register of violent incidents. This register highlighted a progressive increase in in-patient violence over the years. This paper describes research which investigates this rising trend.

Method

The Violent Incidents Register was used to identify 137 psychiatric in-patients who had committed assaults on the ward during 1982. The patients were compared with controls who were matched in terms of age, gender and ward. The case notes of these patients were then analysed and rated according to clinical and demographic criteria.

Results

Of the 137 patients who had committed 470 acts of violence, 72 had been responsible for a total of 405 assaults. The others had committed only one assault each. Of all the assaults, 59% resulted in a detectable injury, 39% in a minor physical injury and 2% in a major physical injury. In most incidents only one person was assaulted. Weapons were used in 19 incidents. The most common victims (i.e. on 78 occasions) were nurses, while other patients were the victims on 53 occasions. The three most serious assaults were committed by men, but there was a slight preponderance of women in other categories. Violent patients were more likely to have a diagnosis of schizophrenia and to have been hallucinating. They were also significantly more likely to be compulsorily detained. Patients in the violent group had had significantly more previous admissions than patients in the control group. Only 13% of violent patients were on their first admission compared with 27% of the control group. The tendency for African–Caribbean patients to commit more serious acts of violence was significant. The incidence rates for delusions, hallucinations, schizophrenia and threatening behaviour were also found to be higher for African–Caribbeans.

Discussion

A substantial increase in violence occurred between the years 1976 and 1984. The increase could not be attributed to an increase in bed numbers. A moderate decrease in violence occurred in 1984 – this could have been because of increased awareness among staff. Patients characterised as violent could best be distinguished by their behavioural characteristics. The proportion of African–Caribbean patients, particularly those in the violent group, was higher than would be expected from numbers in the local population. A striking relationship was found between the ethnicity of a patient and the use of restrictive and compulsory measures. This was most marked in the non-violent control group. The authors suggest that there are particular difficulties in providing a good psychiatric service to African–Caribbean patients and that it cannot be assumed that services based on the needs of the indigenous population will be appropriate for all ethnic subgroups.

Odell, S. M., Surtees, P. G., Wainwright, N. W. J., Commander, M. J. & Sashidharam, S. P. (1997) Determinants of general practitioner recognition of psychological problems in a multi-ethnic inner-city health district. *British Journal of Psychiatry*, **171**, 537–541.

Introduction

Asian patients are said to have psychological problems identified less frequently than their White counterparts, which has been related to greater tendency to somatise or to present with physical problems to the general practitoiner (GP). These authors set out to identify those factors which contribute to a GP's detection of psychological complaints and to examine how these factors influence correct identification of these problems.

Method

One-hundered-and-twenty-five GPs in 66 practices were contacted to provide an estimate of their referrals to psychiatric services in the previous six months, as well as their attitudes to psychological factors in the aetiology of various conditions. Five surgeries were then identified and all patients consulting at non-specialised surgeries during one week were identified and asked to complete a questionnaire. The GP was asked to fill in a consultation form. GHQ–30 was used to measure psychiatric morbidity along with basic socio-demographic details and life-time mental health and current physical health problems. GPs collected information on reasons for consultation, current psychological, social and physical problems, psychiatric diagnosis and current interventions.

Results

Of the 1123 approached, 1039 subjects were able to answer the English language questionnaire but only 908 completed, and GPs completed consultation forms for 951 subjects. Both forms were completed by 833 subjects. Non-responders were more likely to be older and Black within the patient group, and Asian and Black GPs were more likely to be non-responders. GP detection of psychological problems increased with higher scores on GHQ–30 and older patients were more likely to be identified as such. Blacks were underdetected compared with Whites, and Asian GPs were more likely to underdetect. Patients who had social problems or a past history of treated psychiatric disorder were more likely to be detected as having psychological problems. Whites were more likely to be identified correctly as having psychological problems compared with Asian patients. GPs made comparatively fewer psychological diagnoses when physical problems were present.

Clinical factors were the most important factors in determining recognition. GPs' awareness of social problems leads to higher rates of identification of psychological problems. The possibility that more severe cases were identified is reflected by higher scores on GHQ–30. The cultural explanations of mental distress are essential in understanding pathways of care.

Discussion

Bearing in mind that the authors set out to study ethnic differences, it is surprising that they did not use translated versions more universally. As they acknowledge, there remains a problem in identifying psychological or psychiatric conditions if pen and pencil tests are used.

Parkman, S., Davies, S., Leese, M., Phelan, M. & Thornicroft, G. (1997) Ethnic differences in satisfaction with mental health services among representative people with psychosis in south London: PRISM Study 4. *British Journal of Psychiatry*, **171**, 260–264.

Introduction

It has been well-documented that African–Caribbean patients are less likely than White patients to be voluntarily in contact with mental health services, are less likely to have had contact with their general practitioner before admission, have more absences without leave from in-patient wards, have more discharges against medical advice and have fewer regular out-patient attendances. Add to this the higher incidence rates of schizophrenia reported and the higher rates of police referral and forensic sections and it becomes obvious that African–Caribbean patients might find services less satisfactory and relevant to their needs. This paper reports a study in south London investigating levels of satisfaction with mental health services of patients of different ethnic groups diagnosed with psychosis.

Method

A case identification exercise established the prevalence of psychotic disorders in two areas of south London – Nunhead and Norwood. A random sample of psychotic patients was interviewed, in conjunction with their formal and informal carers, using a series of standardised interview schedules. The Verona Service Satisfaction Scale (VSSS), which measures satisfaction with community mental health services, was one of those administered.

Results

Out of the 535 cases of psychosis identified, 202 patients completed the VSSS. Non-responders were not significantly different in terms of socio-demographic or psychiatric profile. Of these, 134 were White and 50 were Black Caribbeans – the rest were excluded from anaysis. There were larger proportions of Black than White patients who were formally detained, younger, female and who had a diagnosis of schizophrenia.

No differences were found in the global level of satisfaction felt. However, Black participants' scores for satisfaction were consistently lower. On one of the individual items measured – satisfaction with specific interventions such as help with side-effects – this lower satisfaction reached significance. When people in each of the ethnic groups were divided into groups born or not born in the UK, the African–Caribbean UK-born patients were found to have significantly lower global satisfaction, which carried over into three of the individual domains tested (skill and behaviour of professionals, efficacy of treatment and specific interventions). All of the groups except the African–Caribbean UK-born patients showed an upward trend in satisfaction with age. Lower satisfaction was found to be associated with the number of admissions a patient had experienced but not the nature of the admission (i.e. whether or not formally detained).

Discussion

The research identifies a complex relationship between satisfaction and ethnicity. The fact that the study was quantitative rather than qualitative prevented the researchers gaining further understanding of why African–Caribbean UK-born patients were more dissatisfied. The authors suggest that there is a vicious cycle of hospital admission, poor satisfaction, less contact with services, poor compliance with medication and relapse, which needs further investigation.

Pipe, R., Bhat, A., Matthews, B. & Hampstead, J. (1991) Section 136 and African/Afro-Caribbean minorities. *International Journal of Social Psychiatry*, **37**, 14–23.

Introduction

Numerous studies have highlighted the over-representation of African and African–Caribbean people compulsorily detained in hospital. This study differs in that it tries to identify specific social and clinical factors that might make racial minorities more vulnerable than others to detention under section 136 of the Mental Health Act.

Method

Social, demographic and clinical data were collected for all referrals under section 136 to Springfield Hospital, south London, in 1996. These details were then compared with local population statistics. For ease of analysis, the sample was divided into three groups by racial origin: European patients, African–Caribbean patients, and a group comprising those from the rest of the New Commonwealth. This last group included people of Asian and African origin.

Results

Ninety-nine patients were admitted under section 136 during the study period. Of these, 64 were White, 21 African–Caribbean, 5 African, 4 Asian, 2 of mixed race, and ethnicity was not known for the rest. A significantly higher proportion of African–Caribbeans were admitted under section 136 than would be expected by local population statistics. This was most marked for African–Caribbeans aged 20–29.

Comparison of the Black (which included African–Caribbean and African patients) and White groups showed that Black patients were more likely to be single, to have been admitted under a 136 section before and, although not statistically significant, to feel that they were not ill. The duty doctors were also twice as likely to record that they were not ill. In addition, Black patients were less likely to have had contact with their general practitioner six months after discharge, although again this difference was not quite significant.

Discussion

As expected, the researchers found an over-representation of African–Caribbeans admitted under section 136 of the Mental Health

Act. In line with previous section 136 research they found that short admissions, high rates of apparent absence of mental illness, high rates of readmission via the same section, high rates of social disadvantage and poor after-care/follow-up arrangements were also features of African–Caribbean admission. In line with more general research into compulsory admission, the following were also features of the sample: they were generally young, single people living alone, who had transient lifestyles and poor social support, and were often unemployed; they had had numerous previous admissions, had diagnoses of either personality disorder or schizophrenia or both, had out-of-hours admissions, had high rates of disturbed behaviours and usually denied being ill. However, unlike in other research studies, both genders featured evenly.

The researchers suggest that to understand why Black people admitted under section tend to be less socially disabled than their White counterparts, there is a need to consider 'institutional racism', especially in relation to understanding how minorities communicate distress and the use of follow-up services.

The researchers also highlight the lack of follow-up information available and recommend further that research is carried out into this area and into the use of alternative social and paramedical support networks.

Prosser, D. (1996) Suicides by burning in England and Wales. *British Journal of Psychiatry*, **168**, 175–182.

Introduction

Suicide by burning (SBB) is a particularly violent and disturbing form of suicide. Epidemiological work has shown that SBB is relatively common in parts of the Middle East and Asia, especially among poorly educated women. Outside the UK, case series investigations of victims admitted to hospital found a high proportion had had previous contact with psychiatric services and that schizophrenia was a more frequent diagnosis than depression. The researchers point out that while SBB is not particularly common in the UK, it is of particular interest because, in 1981, a large case series study in the UK found neither Asian people nor those with a diagnosis of schizophrenia to be over-represented. The fact that more recent epidemiological studies have associated SBB with Asian immigrants, especially women, led the researchers to suggest that the 1981 findings occurred as a result of data from an atypical year.

This study aimed to describe the pattern of SBB in England and Wales since 1981.

Method

All SBB cases in England and Wales registered by the Office of Population Censuses and Surveys in 1991 – the most recent year for which complete data existed – were included in the study. Death certificates, coroners' inquest reports and general practitioners' notes were trawled for socio-demographic information and details on the circumstances of the suicide. Psychiatric information was obtained in the first instance from inquest notes and then followed up in general practitioners' notes. A comparison of SBB and other suicides from 1979 to 1992 was also made to investigate trends in behaviour.

Results

Inquest notes and death certificates of 51 SBB victims were analysed (41 men, 10 women). Thirty-four men and seven women were White and born in the UK; three men were White but born abroad; one man was of mixed race; and three men and three women were first-generation Asian immigrants. So, 30% of women SBB victims were Asian compared with only 7% of men.

In all but one case an accelerant was used. The association between the use of paraffin, as opposed to petrol, and ethnic group (i.e. being Asian) was significant.

In five cases the incident took place intentionally in front of people – this was associated with a diagnosis of personality disorder. In eight cases the victims had been in current contact with psychiatric services, seven had had contact within three months prior to their death and 36 had had no contact within this period. Although 14 of these 36 had had previous, though not recent, contact with mental health services, 15 were known never to have had any contact and a further seven were assumed not to have had. Four people who had not had recent contact with psychiatric services were being treated by their general practitioner for a psychiatric illness and a further four had been treated by their general practitioner in the past. Thirteen of the SBB victims had been previously diagnosed with depression, nine with schizophrenia, four with personality disorder and five with nervous disorders. In the case of a further five people, their diagnosis was not known. Six people were known to be actively psychotic at the time of their deaths and 25 had expressed suicide intent beforehand. Stressors mentioned included: marital problems, redundancy/bankruptcy, bereavement, eviction and the threat of criminal charges.

Discussion

Asian-born women and those with a diagnosis of schizophrenia were found to be over-represented in SBB cases in England and Wales during the period in question. This is in line with most other studies; however, the proportion in contact with psychiatric services was similar to that of suicides as a whole. The author reports that a considerable proportion of cases involved others either as intended victims or as actual witnesses.

Rait, G. & Burns, A (1997) Appreciating background and culture: the South Asian elderly and mental health. *International Journal of Geriatric Psychiatry*, **12**, 973–977.

This editorial comments on several issues referring to South Asian elders which need to be taken into account by the researchers when planning research with these groups. There are key problems which include the definition of ethnicity – whether this is self-ascribed or whether other categories are utilised. Language, history, culture, physical appearance, upbringing, religion and nationality as well as ancestral place of origin need to be considered. In addition, different definitions of 'elderly' are used in different communities. The heterogeneity of individuals within the Indian subcontinent is important in any interpretation of the data. The role of migration in making individuals retain some aspects of their own culture and processes of acculturation are often ignored by researchers. Triple jeopardy of old age, ethnicity and socio-economic deprivation may complicate any interpretation of data. Idioms of distress and ways of communicating distress and perception of symptoms as illness are all key factors in help-seeking by the individuals. The researchers must take into account these factors while planning their studies and interpreting their findings.

Ratan, D., Gandhi D. & Palmer, R. (1998) Eating disorders in British Asians, *International Journal of Eating Disorders*, **24**, 101–105

Introduction

The literature on eating disorders in Asians in the UK is limited and contradictory findings have been reported. This study examines the number and socio-demographic characteristics of Asians presenting to a local eating disorder service.

Method

Asian cases from the case register were identified and ICD–10 research diagnoses were applied. Their social class was determined and rates calculated according to base population.

Results

Twenty-four Asians (23 females, 1 male) were referred in a 10-year period – three did not have an eating disorder. Of 21, 12 (58%) were diagnosed as having bulimia nervosa or atypical bulimia nervosa and 6 (28.6%) had typical or atypical anorexia nervosa. Most belonged to social classes III, IV or V. Crude incidence per year for Asians for anorexia was 0.39 per 100 000 and for bulimia, it was 1.3 per 100 000 (including atypical cases these rates became 0.8 and 1.5 respectively). Over the same period rates for anorexia were 2.0 per 100 000 and bulimia 3.6 per 100 000 for non-Asians.

Clinical characteristics were similar for Asians and non-Asians. Weight concern and fear of fatness were absent. Low rates may be a genuine finding or may reflect a difficulty in obtaining help.

Discussion

The findings were based on retrospective case note study. The authors assume that the base population remained stable over a decade. Small numbers and lack of controls make the findings of limited importance.

Reiss, D. (1996) Abnormal eating attitudes and behaviours in two ethnic groups from a female British urban population. *Psychological Medicine*, **26**, 289–299.

Introduction

Social, cultural, developmental, psychological and biological factors are all thought to play their part in the aetiology of eating disorders. Evidence for eating disorders being a culturally bound syndrome is provided by the apparent rarity of cases seen outside Western cultures. Cultural change has also been implicated as a risk factor – it is thought that the exposure of women from other cultures to Western society may lead to them developing pathological eating attitudes. However, researchers have suggested that the prevalence of eating disorders among Black women living in the West is lower than that of native White populations. The researcher set out to examine the eating attitudes associated with bulimia nervosa in a community sample of second-generation female African–Caribbeans.

Method

All the women who attended four family planning clinics in Tottenham, north London, were asked to take part in the study. (The clinics were chosen for the high proportion of African–Caribbean clients attending.) Three instruments were administered: a specially designed self-report questionnaire to collect demographic information, details of height, weight, eating attitudes/habits and so on; the Bulimic Investigatory Test, Edinburgh (BITE); and the 28-item General Health Questionnaire (GHQ–28). The sample was classified into ethnic groupings and most of those with scores above the threshold for a possible diagnosis of bulimia on the BITE were interviewed further. A number of low-scoring women were also interviewed.

Results

The BITE questionnaire was offered to 475 women under 40 years old, of whom 418 completed it satisfactorily (32.5% African–Caribbean and 45.9% White British women). Of these, 10% of women had a BITE symptom score of 20 or more and/or a severity score of 5 or more, 62% (26) were interviewed – 25% of subjects interviewed were White and 41.7% African–Caribbean. Of the 26 interviewed, six fulfilled the diagnostic criteria for bulimia – one was White British and two were African–Caribbean. All were born in northern Europe.

Comparisons of White British and African–Caribbean subjects showed no significant differences between the two groups in age, marital status, social class and height, although the mean weight of African–Caribbeans was significantly more than that of the White sample. The mean body mass index (BMI) was also significantly greater for African–Caribbeans, as was the mean BITE symptom score. This difference remained significant even when possible interaction effects between the BMI and BITE were taken into account. In terms of the BITE severity score, 12.5% of African–Caribbean subjects and 5.7% of White subjects were over the cut-off score. This difference was significant. There was no significant difference found between the two groups on any of the GHQ subscales. The symptom profiles of the two groups on BITE highlighted three questions where a significantly higher proportion of African–Caribbeans scored positively (i.e. answered 'Yes'). These were: 'If you overeat do you feel guilty?', 'Do you feel a failure if you break your diet once?' and 'Would you say that food dominated your life?'. Differences in the groups' responses to a further three questions tended towards significance: 'Do you eat sensibly in front of others and make up in private?', 'Are your eating habits what you would consider normal?' and 'Do you ever experience overpowering urges to eat and eat and eat?'.

Comparisons within the African–Caribbean sample by birthplace were made. A significant difference was found in age and marital status – those born abroad were older and more likely to be married. No other significant differences were found.

Discussion

The level of dysfunctional eating attitudes found among African–Caribbean subjects was significantly higher than that found among the White British subjects. The results, the author says, demolishes the myth that the Black population has a low level of eating problems. The problems in using instruments standardised on Western populations on other cultural groups are acknowledged. The author also highlights problems in assuming that the findings, based on this specific sample, can be generalised to the wider population.

Sellwood, W. & Tarrier, N. (1994) Demographic factors associated with extreme non-compliance in schizophrenia. *Social Psychiatry and Psychiatric Epidemiology*, **29**, 172–177.

Introduction

Neuroleptic medication is seen as the most effective treatment for managing the symptoms of schizophrenia and for preventing relapse. However, studies looking at compliance with medication have estimated non-compliance rates of between 10% and 76%. Research into factors associated with non-compliance (often producing conflicting results) has investigated side-effects, type of symptoms, approach to service delivery, psychological factors such as beliefs about schizophrenia and the consequences of the illness, and demographic details. This paper attempts to clarify whether ethnicity is associated with non-compliance.

Method

The records of patients discharged from central Manchester's Department of Psychiatry between January 1989 and December 1991 were examined and details of patients with schizophrenic disorders or schizoaffective disorders were extracted. Forty-three patients who persistently refused all maintenance neuroleptic medication were identified, along with 213 patients who were only partially compliant.

Results

Of the 256 patients identified, 71 were of African–Caribbean origin. There were 108 women and 145 men. The mean age of the sample was 36.4 years (range 17–70 years). Each patient on average spent 116.2 days in hospital before discharge (range 1–1973 days). The very non-compliant (VNC) patients were significantly different from the other group. They were more likely to be African–Caribbean, male and to have had more hospital admissions – although during the three years of the study they spent significantly less time in hospital. African–Caribbean men were more likely to be non-compliant than African–Caribbean women but no such difference was seen with non-African–Caribbean men and women. Male African–Caribbeans were significantly more likely to be in the VNC group than their non-African–Caribbean counterparts. This was not the case for African–Caribbean women. African–Caribbeans in the VNC group were also significantly younger than their non-African–Caribbean counterparts. The women in this group tended to be older than men. Thus ethnic origin was a significant predictor of non-compliance, as was gender but to a lesser extent. Age, however, was not a significant predictor of compliance.

Discussion

Patient compliance ratings were based on their consultants' recollections of what happened – this may have biased the results. It should also be noted that while gender and ethnicity were found to be significant predictors of compliance, the effects of these two factors were very small. Differences in the subjective experience of medication, dosage, aggression and involuntary status were all considered as possible reasons for African–Caribbean men being almost twice as likely to be in the VNC group. However only the last two of these factors were thought to be of significance. The authors point out that ethnic factors involved in determining compliance are complex and that socio-economic status, a variable that has been shown in other studies to be related to compliance, was not included in this investigation.

Shah, A., Lindesay, J. & Jagger, C. (1997) Is the diagnosis of dementia stable over time among elderly immigrant Gujuratis in the United Kingdom (Leicester)? *International Journal of Geriatric Psychiatry*, **13**, 440–444.

Introduction

Following on from Lindesay *et al*'s (1997) study Gujurati elderly subjects who had been diagnosed as having dementia were followed up 27 months later. In the original study 11 patients had been diagnosed as having dementia on standard mini-mental state examination.

Method

Seven subjects were alive at follow-up and were interviewed, and information was obtained on another three through their carers.

Results

Six of the seven subjects alive at follow-up showed further cognitive decline whereas the seventh subject was thought not to have dementia at follow-up. There were three cases of Alzheimer's disease, two of vascular dementia and one of mixed dementia.

The dementia cases had a cognitive decline and the causes of dementia vary as they do in other populations.

Discussion

In spite of small numbers, the study highlights the possibility that dementia can be recognised across cultures using suitable and appropriate translations.

Shaw, C. M., Creed, F., Babbs, C., Guthrie, E. A. & Tommenson, B. (1996) Referral of Asian patients to a GI clinic. *Journal of Psychosomatic Research*, **41**, 473–479.

Introduction

There is a similar level of psychiatric disorder among UK Asian and White general practice attendees, and yet South Asians are more likely to present somatic symptoms and less likely to seek help for psychological problems. In such cases, general practitioners often miss psychological distress; consequently, a large proportion of people attending out-patient clinics with medically unexplained symptoms are thought to have a psychiatric disorder. For example, research has shown that people with a functional bowel disorder are two to three times more likely than those suffering an organic bowel disease to have a psychiatric disorder. This study compares the level of psychiatric disorder among patients of South Asian and White European origin attending gastrointestinal (GI) clinics.

Method

Referrals to the weekly out-patient and endoscopy clinics of two consultants specialising in GI disorders and based in Rochdale (an area with a high Asian population) were scrutinised. Over a six-month period all newly referred Asian patients aged between 16 and 65 were recruited to the study, along with the next presenting White European patient of similar age, gender and diagnosis. The patients were divided into groups according to ethnic origin (Asian or White European) and diagnosis (functional or organic). Further demographic information, duration and severity of symptoms, along with the psychiatric status of each patient, were all rated.

Results

There were 36 Asian and 36 White patients recruited for the study. Each group had equal numbers of men and women, a mean age of 39 years and a similar range of GI symptoms.

Significant demographic differences were found. Asian patients had lower levels of formal education and more children both living at home and in total. Asian women were more likely to work exclusively in the home.

The duration and severity of symptoms were found to be significantly lower for Asian patients with a functional diagnosis compared with White patients in the same situation. The trend was for Asian patients to have had symptoms for longer, although this difference was not quite significant, and neither was the statistical difference in the numbers felt to have a definite psychiatric disorder – 23% of Asian and 42% of White patients. The diagnosis given to patients in all but one of these patients (who was given a diagnosis of anxiety) was depression. There was no difference in the prevalence of psychiatric disorder among Asians with functional or organic diagnoses. This contrasts with the comparison of the two White groups, where patients with a functional diagnosis were more likely to be categorised as having a psychiatric disorder.

Discussion

In line with previous studies, the research found higher rates of unrecognised depression and anxiety in Asian patients; however, the original hypothesis that there would be a greater prevalence of psychiatric disorder in Asian patients with somatic symptoms compared with their White counterparts had to be rejected. These findings, in conjunction with the lower severity of symptoms in Asian patients, lead the authors to suggest that general practitioners have a lower threshold for referring Asian patients than White patients. The relatively high proportion of White patients who had been through higher education also suggests bias on the part of general practitioners.

The researchers conclude by stating that the large numbers of Asian patients with a functional GI disorder needs to be recognised and effective ways of assessing such patients developed. The relatively small numbers of subjects and the use of interpreters are recognised as some of the limitations of the study. Further research into pathways to care, prevalence of functional disorders among ethnic groups and prevalence of somatic symptoms is recommended.

Sheth, H., Dziewulski, P. & Settle, J. A. D. (1994) Self-inflicted burns: a common way of suicide in the Asian population. A 10-year retrospective study. *Burns,* **20,** 334–335.

Introduction

Suicide by burning is relatively uncommon in the West, more usually occurring among Asian and African women. This study was an investigation of both demographic and outcome data on patients admitted to the Yorkshire Regional Burns Unit over a 10-year period.

Method

A survey of patients admitted to the unit between March 1983 and March 1993 revealed 20 who had been admitted with a suicidal burn injury. Information about age, percentage area burned, areas involved, marital status, number of children, psychiatric history and socio-economic status was collected, along with mortality and morbidity data.

Results

Of the 20 patients admitted (8.54% of total admissions) with a history of suicidal burns, 3 were male and 17 female. Of the female patients,

14 (70%) were of Asian origin – none had a psychiatric history. The three other females and all three males were White, and all had a psychiatric history. Ages ranged from 19 to 43 years (mean 28.8 years). Of the Asian women, 6 (43%) were between 20 and 25 years old. All the Asian women were married, were housewives and had two to six children. Most had migrated to the UK after their marriage. Most had poured kerosene on to their clothes before setting light to themselves. Burns covered between 25% and 99% of their body. Burns were typically located on the face, neck, trunk and arms of the women. Of these 14 women, nine died and five survived.

Discussion

The research shows that self-inflicted burns are indeed a relatively common form of suicide among Asian women. The authors highlight the relatively high rates of suicide in young Asian women both within Asia and in countries where they have settled. They point out that the causes of self-injury by Asian women reported from studies both within and outside Asia are similar. (Causes reported include: a culture that puts a premium on academic and economic success; stigma attached to failure; and authority of elders coupled with expected unquestioning compliance from younger family members.) Migration itself, therefore, cannot be the cause of these high suicide rates, although it may exacerbate the situation. The researchers highlight the need for appropriate counselling services organised by people familiar with Asian languages and culture (i.e. from within their local communities).

Silveira, E. R. & Ebrahim, S. (1998) A comparison of mental health among minority ethnic elders and whites in East and North London. *Age and Ageing,* **27,** 375–383.

Introduction

The authors emphasise that morbidity rates are a better indicator of population health patterns and, by extension, of the existence of health inequalities. They set out to compare rates of various psychiatric disorders across different ethnic groups, to compare these with Whites and to explore the underlying reasons for differential rates and whether these are associated with life satisfaction.

Method

Using a range of methods such as snowballing techniques, luncheon clubs and general practice surgery registers, subjects were recruited for the study. The self-rating scale of symptoms of anxiety and depression, which focuses on symptomatology in the past week, was used and life satisfaction was measured using a 13-item version of the life satisfaction scale. Appropriate translations were used for different groups.

Results

Seventy-two Somalis (60 men, 12 women), 75 Bengalis (52 men, 23 women) and 127 whites (60 men, 67 women) in East London and 41 Gujuratis (21 men, 20 women) and 63 Whites (30 men, 33 women) in north London were interviewed. North London Whites were the oldest (mean age 70.2) and Bengalis the youngest (63.6). White patients were the least likely to be married and 91% Bengalis were married. Disability was higher among the youngest. A quarter of Somalis were depressed compared with 77% of Bengalis and 2% of Gujuratis. Correlation coefficients showed a significant correlation between medical problems and disability among Bengalis and East London Whites only.

Disability among Somalis was low, although ideas that disability constituted moral weakness or lack of faith in God were identified. A negative correlation between age and depression was found in some groups suggesting that their idioms of distress are different.

Discussion

The study shows some interesting differences across ethnic groups but there are serious methodological problems. Also, the Bengalis mean age is well below 65 suggesting a bias in sample selection.

Silveira, E. R. & Shah, E. (1998) Social determinants of psychiatric morbidity and well-being in immigrant elders and whites in East London. *International Journal of Geriatric Psychiatry*, **13**, 801–812.

Introduction

The impact of migration on mental health varies on both physical and psychological fronts. In older individuals, the initial effects of selection and migration ususally pass and studies often neglect social determinants of mental health and well-being in elderly people. A triple jeopardy of ageing, belonging to an ethnic minority and mental illness will influence help- seeking.

Method

Immigrants were recruited through snowballing, luncheon clubs and general practice registers in East London. A standardised questionnaire translated into appropriate languages was used to collect information on demographic, social and health factors and satisfaction with services provided. Anxiety and depression were measured using a self-rating scale of anxiety and depression, and life satisfaction using a life satisfaction index. Social factors included information on housing problems, lack of family support and personal difficulties.

Results

Seventy-two Somalis (60 men, 12 women), 75 Bengalis (52 men, 23 women) were the subjects. Bengalis had the youngest mean age, were least likely to be living alone and were most likely to be living in poor housing. They were also most likely to have one or more medical problems as well as physical disability. The Bengalis had the highest prevalence (77%) of scores in the depressed range, whereas in the other two groups the prevalence was 25%. Social factors and physical health factors were the most significant risk factors for a low life satisfaction index.

Discussion

The authors suggest that differential mental health rates are related to social factors. Their findings on Bengali subjects are intriguing, and cultural idioms of distress may contribute to excess but cannot really explain such a high differential.

The methodology of recruitment of subjects is weak and remains a source of bias. The gender difference in the sample needs to be taken into account when interpreting the data.

Singh, S. P., Croudace, T., Beck, A. and Harrison, G. (1998) Perceived ethnicity and the risk of compulsory admission. *Social Psychiatry and Psychiatric Epidemiology*, **33**, 39–44.

Introduction

The reports on excess of compulsory admissions in patients of African–Caribbean ethnicity have suggested several possible reasons for this excess, although rates among first onset cases of schizophrenia have not been shown to be as high. The authors set out to study the risk of compulsory admission among different ethnic groups.

Method

All consecutive admissions to acute admission wards in Nottingham over a six-month period were approached to take part in the study. Information was obtained on reasons for admission, symptom profile, evidence of risk and clinical diagnosis.

Results

Of 481 patients admitted, data on ethnicity and Mental Health Act status were available on 464 and 461 cases respectively. Complete data were available on 417 cases of whom 91 (22%) were admitted compulsorily. Asian patients were more likely to be male, younger and less likely than their counterparts to be compulsorily detained or have a diagnosis of psychosis. The authors then went on to exclude Asians because they were said not to differ on rates of compulsory admission. Black Caribbeans were more likely to have psychosis and 43.2% of admissions were compulsory compared with 18.8% for Whites. Compulsorily detainment was significantly related to having a diagnosis of psychosis, being unemployed and being considered at risk of violence. These factors remained related to ethnicity and compulsorily admission.

Black patients are at an increased risk of being compulsorily admitted to acute wards with an adjusted odds ration of 2.16. Perception of risk of violence is an important factor in the decision to detain patients irrespective of their ethnicity.

Discussion

Admissions are dictated by a series of factors. The study did not control for alternative handling of different ethnic groups. By excluding Asians, the authors weakened their study and the question of perceived ethnicity has not been adequately answered.

Sugarman, P. A. & Craufurd, D. (1994) Schizophrenia in the Afro-Caribbean community. *British Journal of Psychiatry*, **164**, 474–480.

Introduction

A series of studies have reported higher rates of schizophrenia among Caribbean-born people in the UK. Attempting to find the cause of the outbreak will help to answer important questions about the aetiology of the disease. Genetic factors are known to play their part, but a significant role is also played by non-genetic factors. The most widely accepted model concerning the aetiology of schizophrenia is a multi-factorial one. This proposes that when the combined effect of genetic and environmental factors exceed some threshold, individuals develop symptoms of schizophrenia. The authors suggest that the question of whether or not the high prevalence rates experienced by second-generation African–Caribbeans are due to environment factors can be answered by investigating the rates of illness that exist in relatives. If, they say, genetic factors are not the important ones, then rates among relatives should be lower for African–Caribbeans than Whites. This study investigated this hypothesis by comparing rates of illness among first-degree relatives of patients diagnosed with schizophrenia.

Method

The case notes were examined of in-patients with schizophrenia admitted over a seven-year period to hospitals within the catchment area of a central Manchester health district. Patients meeting Research Diagnostic Criteria for schizophrenia, of African–Caribbean origin, and the next White patient of similar gender and age, were included in the study. The majority of patients in the control group were of Irish origin.

Results

Thirty-six African–Caribbean and 39 White patients were recruited. A family history of schizophrenia, schizoaffective disorder or unspecified psychosis was found for 50% of the African–Caribbean patients and 33% of the White patients. However, this difference was not statistically significant. African–Caribbeans born in the UK were found to be more likely to have a family history than those who were not, but this result could have been influenced by difficulty in obtaining accurate information about relatives abroad. The research also found that first-degree relatives of African–Caribbean men had a significantly higher risk of the disease than the relatives of women. This difference was even more marked when only UK-born African–Caribbeans were considered.

Discussion

From these results it appears that schizophrenia in the African–Caribbean community is no less familial than in the White population. The authors suggest that although their findings were not consistent with their original hypothesis (i.e. that genetic predisposition was less important in the aetiology of schizophrenia in the Black UK population) the results also do not support the notion that the higher prevalence is due to greater genetic vulnerability. It is proposed that the increased rates are due to as yet undetermined environmental factors.

Suhail, K. & Cochrane, R. (1998) Seasonal variations in hospital admissions for affective disorders by gender and ethnicity. *Social Psychiatry & Psychiatric Epidemiology*, **33**, 211–217.

Introduction

Seasonality has been linked with several psychiatric disorders but systematic studies are few and far between. The authors set out to study seasonality of admissions for psychiatric disorders by ethnicity. They hypothesised that admissions for depression would peak in winter in all groups, but that the Asians would show a greater frequency of depressive episodes.

Method

Using a retrospective case note study method they traced 965 case notes – a total of 676 patients contributing to 903 admissions. Three main categories of ethnicity – Asian, White and Black were used. ICD–10 diagnoses were broadly divided into mood disorders and non-mood disorders. Local monthly climatic data were collected.

Results

Of 903 patients, 596 were White (307 men, 289 women), 163 Asian (115 men, 48 women) and 144 Black (79 men, 65 women). The mean age for Asians was significantly lower and Asians were most likely to have diagnosis of schizophrenia. There were no significant seasonal effects on overall admissions or admissions due to non-mood disorders. However, only women showed a significant seasonal variation in the frequency of admissions for depression with the incidence being highest in winter. When seasonal effects for bipolar admissions were examined separately for men and women, women showed a summer peak. Only the Asian group showed significant seasonality in depression, with a greater number of depressive

episodes in winter. Multiple regression analyses using monthly climatic data showed that climatic factors did not contribute significantly to the monthly variations in total admissions.
Significant seasonal peaks were found for mood disorder admissions but not for total admissions. Seasonal peaks were opposite for depression and bipolar disorder. The winter peak for depressive admissions accords with some previous reports. The effect of ethnicity was notable only for depression.

Discussion

Although it is the first study to look at patterns of seasonality, mood disorder, gender and ethnicity, it relies on case notes. Admissions of less serious cases may have been unlikely, thus the study does not represent true incidence.

Takei, N., Persaud, R., Woodruff, P., Brockington, I. & Murray, R. M. (1998) First episodes of psychosis in Afro-Caribbean and White people. An 18-year follow-up population-based study. *British Journal of Psychiatry*, **172**, 147–153.

Introduction

Long-term outcome studies of African–Caribbean patients show a varied picture. The authors set out to follow up a series of African–Caribbean and White patients with psychosis diagnosed in 1973–1974.

Method

Originally all first admissions from the Camberwell area were identified in 1973–1974 and included 34 African–Caribbean and 54 White British-born people. The follow-up was 18 years later. The subjects were examined using the Present State Examination, Social Adjustment Scale and Global Assessment Scale.

Results

Of the 54 Whites, 51 were traced – three refused an interview and two had died. Of the 34 African–Caribbeans, all were traced – two refused and two had died. Additional information was obtained from general practitioners, hospital staff and case notes. Thus the sample consisted of 49 Whites and 32 African–Caribbeans. The mean age at first admission was significantly younger for African–Caribbeans who were also more likely to come from lower socio-economic backgrounds. The diagnostic consistency of schizophrenia was slightly higher for African–Caribbeans than for Whites. The African–Caribbeans had a median length of admissions for 255 days compared with 89 days for Whites and this was associated with ethnicity and diagnosis, not age of onset. Experience of compulsory admissions also varied according to ethnicity and diagnosis. African–Caribbeans had significantly worse outcomes in "symptom related dysfunctioning and limited leisure activity", which was not influenced by paternal social class or age of onset.

Diagnostic consistency and follow-up presence of psychosis were broadly similar in the two groups. The most striking differences were in the psychiatric care experienced by the two groups: African–Caribbeans had had more frequent admissions, longer hospitalisations and more compulsory treatment. There was no evidence to suggest that African–Caribbeans were more likely to experience brief reactive psychoses.

Discussion

This study is the first to provide a long-term outcome of psychoses in African–Caribbean and White patients from the same catchment area. Other social factors such as socio-economic deprivation and racial hassles may have influenced the outcome of African–Caribbean patients more adversely.

Thornicroft, G., Meadows, G. & Politi, P. (1992) Is 'cannabis psychosis' a distinct category? *European Psychiatry*, **7**, 277–282.

Introduction

Cannabinoids have long been associated with psychosis. However, some have suggested that there should be a distinct diagnostic category of 'cannabis psychosis'. This study investigated the validity of such a claim.

Method

The medical records were examined of in-patients at the Royal Bethlem and Maudsley Hospital, admitted between 1976 and 1986 with psychosis linked to cannabis consumption. Patients included in the study were between 16 and 65 years old and had given a urine sample which tested positive for cannabis sometime during their admission. Information about these patients was compared with data from other patients admitted during the same 10-year period who had a non-organic psychotic disorder. The Syndrome Check-List, which uses case note information to rate 25 syndromes, was applied.

Results

The two groups of patients were not significantly different in terms of gender or age on index admission. There were significantly more African–Caribbeans in the group with cannabis-associated psychosis than in the other group.

The researchers found that 21 of the syndromes investigated were significantly more common in the group of cannabis users. These were the syndromes related to coherence of speech and agitation. Case note and primary discharge diagnosis were also investigated, but no significant differences were found between the two patient groups.

Discussion

No clear pattern of symptoms appears to distinguish the group of cannabis users from the non-cannabis users – although the researchers recommend caution should be used when interpreting the data from a retrospective study such as this. Their findings, however, do suggest that evidence for a non-organic 'cannabis psychosis' as a distinct diagnostic category is weak.

Van Os, J., Takei, N., Castle, D., Wessely, S., Der, G., MacDonald, A. M. & Murray, R. M. (1996) The incidence of mania: time trends in relation to gender and ethnicity. *Social Psychiatry and Psychiatric Epidemiology*, **31**, 129–136.

Introduction

Numerous researchers have identified African–Caribbeans in the UK as having a higher risk of developing schizophrenia than the White population. The researchers investigate whether this increased risk extends to mania. Conflicting reports exist about changes in incidence rates for mania in the 1970s and '80s – particularly in respect of ethnicity. These differing results may have been due to confounding factors such as changes in diagnostic habits and the inclusion of second-generation African–Caribbeans in the comparison group. The authors highlight the importance of investigation because of the implications for service provision and theories of aetiology. This study explores time trends in incidence rates and their ethnic distribution in an area of south London.

Method

The Camberwell Cumulative Psychiatric Case Register provides information about Camberwell residents who had their first contact with psychiatric services between 1964 and 1984. The research sample included patients on the register with a diagnosis of mania or hypomania. The information in patients' case notes was used to obtain a further diagnosis according to Research Diagnostic Criteria. Demographic information about the sample was collected and compared with data for the general population of the area from the 1961, 1971 and 1981 censuses. Incidence rates for mania and mania with schizomania were calculated for the years 1965–69, 1970–74, 1975–79 and 1980–84.

Results

The trend was for an increase in incidence rates for both mania and mania with schizomania over the whole period of the study, 1965–84. Overall incidence rates were similar for both genders but the increase in incidence rates was significant only for females. The proportion of Caribbean-born patients with mania was eight times higher than UK-born patients in the period 1965–69 and between three and five times higher in the 1970s. In the years 1980–84, the rate of mania for all African–Caribbeans, including those born in the UK, was four times higher than that for all other ethnic groups combined (the majority of whom were White). Among those with mania, African–Caribbeans were significantly more likely to fulfil the criteria for schizophrenia. After corrections were made for differences in the age distributions of ethnic groups in the general population of the catchment area, African–Caribbeans were found to have incidence rates for mania with schizomania over three times that of their White counterparts, while the rate for mania was more than double that of their White counterparts.

Investigation of patients with a first onset of depression showed that there was equal probability of patients who subsequently developed mania being born in the UK or the Caribbean. Contrary to expectations, African–Caribbeans in this group were more likely to receive follow-up diagnoses of mania and psychosis, especially schizophrenia. African–Caribbeans were also less likely to receive a subsequent diagnosis of neurosis or personality disorder.

Discussion

The difficulties inherent in using census data to estimate incidence rates make it impossible to attribute, with any certainty, the increased rates of mania found to changes in the ethnic composition of the local area. In any case, the size of the increase indicates that there is an increase independent of any growth in the African–Caribbean population. Other studies have found higher rates of mania in a variety of ethnic minority groups. It may be that the common sources of stress experienced by ethnic minorities are important determinants of incidence rates. Consideration was given to other explanations for the increased rates of mania found, across the whole of the local population, but changes in the gender, age and socio-economic structure of the area were not felt to be large enough to account for the results.

Wittkower, E. D. (1970) Transcultural psychiatry in the Caribbean: past, present, and future. *American Journal of Psychiatry*, **127**, 162–166.

Introduction

The Caribbean islands are of special interest because of their cultural diversity. Furthermore, they include regions in widely different stages of economic development and political status. Despite the many differences, however, their common heritage of slavery, African origin and plantation economy means that the islands have much in common. Within the islands there also exists a diversity of household structures. Apart from the nuclear family (which is still common), of great importance is the matrifocal household – that is one where women predominate and a male sexual partner is not permanently present. The author believes the psychological consequences of this arrangement to include: "deep attachments of men to their mothers, uneasy relationships with other women, potency doubts resulting in promiscuity and ostentatious displays of virility".

The author reviews culturally focused psychiatric research carried out in the Caribbean. He investigates the frequency distribution and symptomatology of mental disorders, the reasons for differences in psychiatric disorders between Caribbean and other cultures, and specific problems encountered by psychiatrists practising in the area.

Research review

Traditionally, psychiatrists from outside the area have concerned themselves with phenomena not found in their own cultures, such as voodoo ceremonies and possession states. Indigenous psychiatrists, on the other hand, have focused on more practical problems, such as alcoholism. No large-scale epidemiological studies had been carried out regarding the incidence of mental illness in the Caribbean. But some small studies have had interesting results. For example, a survey of untreated mental illness reported an unusually high rate of mild schizophrenia in women and a low rate of psychotic depression in men when compared with the US. The researchers pointed to genetic, sociocultural and psychocultural factors as possible reasons for their findings.

Attempts, in the main, to relate mental illness to family structure have not met with much success. Some have argued that matrifocal families create a sense of insecurity. The 1960 census of mental hospitals in the Caribbean revealed that a higher proportion of male patients than females who were single and unattached were suffering from functional psychosis. It has been argued that this is because Caribbean males are less secure and less able to bear their loneliness.

With regard to the distribution of disorders in the region, the reviewer states that malnutrition, chronic infectious diseases and parasitic diseases contribute significantly to the course of psychiatric disorders in the Caribbean. A profile of the common disorders is as follows: the paranoid form of schizophrenia, often associated with delirium and catatonia, was found to be the most common; the level of alcoholism was found to be high and increasing on some islands; manic depression was a feature, but patients were much more likely to be admitted to hospital as a result of manic excitement than depression; acute transitory psychotic states, usually precipitated by stressful life events, were also common in the region (the contention is that they constitute a culturally accepted means of escape from intolerable emotional conflict for those whose egos are weak and poorly constructed); and finally possession states, a particular phenomenon of the region, are thought to be a cultural variant of the hypnotic state. There is great debate as to whether possession is predominantly culturally sanctioned, an inherited form of neurosis or something different altogether that needs further investigation.

The role of the native healer versus that of medically trained psychiatrists in treating the mentally ill is also an area of debate.

Author index

Compiled by CAROLINE SHEARD

Subject index

Compiled by CAROLINE SHEARD